The
PSYCHIATRIC
HOSPITAL

Context,
Values, and
Therapeutic Process

The
PSYCHIATRIC
HOSPITAL

Context,
Values, and
Therapeutic Process

by

Henry L. Lennard, Ph.D.

in collaboration with

Alexander Gralnick, M. D.

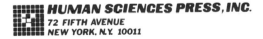 **HUMAN SCIENCES PRESS, INC.**
72 FIFTH AVENUE
NEW YORK, N.Y. 10011

Library of Congress Cataloging-in-Publication Data

Lennard, Henry L.
 The psychiatric hospital.

 Bibliography: p. 211
 Includes index.
 1. Psyciatric hospital care. 2. Psychoses—
Treatment. 3. Personality, Disorders of—Treatment.
I. Gralnick, Alexander, 1912–   . II. Title.
[DNLM: 1. Hospitals, Psychiatric—trends.
2. Psychotherapy—methods. 3. Psychotherapy—trends.
WM 420 L567p]
RC439.L46   1986   362.2'1
ISBN 0-89885-297-8

This book is affectionately dedicated to Dr. Alexander Gralnick, whose work provided the stimulus for it.

Alexander Gralnick and his colleagues have been engaged, over the past 30 years, in designing and developing a unique social and physical treatment context. The therapeutic program of High Point Hospital exemplifies the essential features of social therapy as described in this book.

CONTENTS

ACKNOWLEDGEMENTS

Dr. Suzanne Crowhurst-Lennard, Ph.D. (Architecture) is primarily responsible for the section on "The Physical Setting as a Therapeutic Modality." The book incorporates sections of an earlier report written in collaboration with Dr. Donald Ransom.

"I am a part of all that I have met," says Tennyson's *Ulysses*. I have indeed been fortunate that my work on therapeutic processes has brought me into collaborative relations with many thoughtful and innovative clinicians. I have worked with Nathan Ackerman, Arnold Bernstein, Donald Bloch, Leon Epstein, Alexander Gralnick, Donald

Jackson, Stephen Kempster, Helen Meyers, and Harley Shands. Over the years I have also benefitted from the work of many colleagues and friends: Matthias C. Angermeyer, Robert Bales, Howard Becker, Gregory Bateson, Albert Jonsen, Theodore Lidz, Robert Merton, Frederick Meyers, Peter Novak, Ivan Boszormenyi-Nagy, Johann Jurgen Rohde, Jurgen Ruesch, Nevitt Sanford, John Spiegel, Anselm Strauss, and Otto Allen Will. Having been exposed to a variety of intellectual disciplines and theoretical frameworks, I have been challenged by Butterfield's statement that "of all forms of mental activity the most difficult to induce . . . is the art of handling the same bundle of data as before but placing them in a new system of relations with one another by giving them a different framework." In this connection, I wish to express my gratitude to Mr. Philip Sapir who supported my work at the interface of clinical practice and behavioral science, while President of the Grant Foundation.

Though one of the first social scientists to be invited to be a member of the American College of Neuropsychopharmacology, an interdisciplinary group devoted to the exploration of the role of drugs in psychiatric treatment, I have, over the years, become troubled by the behavioral and ethical risks connected with the mass deployment of this modality. Though still deeply impressed with Freud's vision and the contribution of psychoanalysis, I have come nonetheless to agree with Philip Rieff that the "triumph of the therapeutic" is not always a blessing. And finally, though I had been very active at the beginnings of the family therapy movement—as a consultant to emerging family therapy enterprises both on the east and west coasts—I no longer share the fervor that prevails among family system theorists who seem to have exchanged a faith in "systems" for a belief in the "unconscious." An analysis of current conceptions of mental disorder and my own preference for a multi-faceted yet benign model are presented in the appendix on A Conception of Mental Disorder.

As my friend and teacher Harley Shands used to say when told the wonders of new therapeutic, religious, or social movement: "I was Saved when I was 14." I too was never a true believer! If there is an ideology I confess to, then it is to that expressed by Harry Stack Sullivan: "We are all much more simply human than otherwise, be we happy and successful, contented and detached, miserable and mentally disordered or whatever."

Henry L. Lennard, Ph.D.

PREFACE

The revolution in psychiatric treatment methods initiated by Freud at the turn of the 19th century gradually came to dominate the thinking of most psychiatric practitioners by the middle of the 20th century, whether they worked in their offices or in hospitals. The assumption that underlay this thinking was that the mental disorders that human beings develop are due to repressed conflicts or faulty defense mechanisms; hence, therapeutic emphasis was usually placed on intensive efforts to "uncover" the intra-psychic distortions and defenses interfering with the individual's ability to cope more effectively. The environment was treated more or less as a "given."

In some psychoanalytic circles, this conception was carried over into the treatment of the "functional" psychoses, and particularly of schizophrenia. Countless hours and years were spent analyzing the meaning of the behavior, delusions, and hallucinations of schizophrenic patients, on the assumption that enabling them to understand what they were doing defensively and intrapsychically would ultimately lead to their cure. The major emphasis in all of this was on increasing the understanding of the individual and on eliminating his "repressions." Freud's famous dictum: "Where id was, there shall ego be," was translated in practice to mean that the more uncovering of repressed material that could be brought into consciousness, the greater would be the ultimate health of the individual.

Beginning in the latter half of the 20th century, however, a new point of view began to make itself felt in the approach to mental disorder that constituted a psychiatric revolution of almost equal importance to that initiated by Freud. This placed the locus of psychopathology not just within the intrapsychic mechanisms of the individual, but rather in the nature of his interpersonal relationships, and in the dynamic interaction between the intrapsychic dynamics of the individual and the sociodynamics of his surrounding medium. Thus, the locus of psychopathology was no longer sought within the disordered mind of the individual, but rather within the distorted *system* of his interpersonal and social relationships, and the impact of these disordered relationships on the individual's developmental processes.

This shift in conceptualization has led to major changes in the way psychotherapy, both within and out of the mental hospital, has begun to be conducted. In individual psychotherapy, emphasis is no longer placed only on the "uncovering" process, or on the giving of "insights," but also on an understanding of the reality factors that have led to the decompensatory process and of modifying them wherever possible. Moreover, the therapeutic process itself is no longer conceived of as one in which a therapist transmits understanding to a patient, but rather as a dynamic interaction between two individuals, in which the therapist's empathic and caring responsiveness and benign guidance both overtly and covertly play a major contributory role.

Within mental hospitals, also, the emphasis has shifted from reductionistic approaches that were primarily biological or psychological, to ones that consider the entire bio-psycho-social system involved in the patient's psychopathology. As the authors of the present volume indicate, this encompasses an awareness even of the relationship of structural and architectural elements to the total therapeutic process. The reader will find the present volume to be a mature reflection of the new ways of thinking about the inpatient treatment of seriously disturbed individuals, and particularly of those with severe character disorders and functional psychoses. The authors make no pretense that this work is a final statement. Rather, throughout the book they delineate the way their thinking has evolved over the years, and is still continuing to evolve. They also recognize that many questions remain to be resolved. Nevertheless, for clinicians who have occasion to hospitalize patients with such disorders, and for the many thousands of psychiatrists and other mental health workers who are engaged in the complex task of treating such patients, this book can serve as a valuable guide to illuminate some of the perplexing problems that they may encounter on their challenging journey.

Judd Marmor, M.D.

PREFACE

This stimulating book has struck a number of responsive chords in me. It has been two decades since a team of us studied psychiatric ideologies and the work of staffs at the Psychosomatic and Psychiatric Institute of Michael Reese and the Chicago State Hospital in Chicago. Then, the predominant modes of treatment were the psychosomatic and the somatic, with milieu therapy just beginning to appear in American hospitals. In the two decades since, of course, there have been striking changes in psychiatric thinking, research, treatments and in the institutions; but to an outsider sociologist like me, an equally striking feature of the mental health scene is the evidence of continued strong disagreement over some basic issues bearing on etiology, treatment and treatment outcomes.

One way to read this book is to regard it, as I did, as a careful scrutiny by an insider-outsider (Lennard) who, in dialogue with a psychiatrist-director (Gralnick), has given us a valuable account of the workings out of one approach to treatment process and the organization of a psychiatric treatment setting. Dr. Lennard has been *specific* in tracing out the elements of this approach-in-operation. This is what gives conviction to his study, and persuades us that his observations and interpretations support this institution's claims that treatment is much more than physician to patient interaction, or more than standard milieu approaches insist upon. Lennard focuses us on the total institutional gestalt, including even the details of its spatial arrangements and the predominant interactional patterns among everyone in the institution—patients and staff alike.

Among the kinds of interactions described in this book are treatment modalities conceptualized by Lennard as forms of therapeutic work. Here his perspective comes closest to my own. Activities which involve tasks and task performances lend themselves readily to a work perspective, including concepts of division of labor, accountability, and the coordination or articulation of tasks. Lennard makes us understand some of this with his isolation of types of work like attentional work, informational work, achieving membership (a particularly astute interpretation), trust work and competence work. He also underlines what I discovered myself from the study of acute care hospitals, that patients are workers too, and that to understand the effects of treatments we have to look at their parts in the total drama.

We are also reminded, forcefully, that schizophrenia is one of the chronic illnesses, presently incurable.

Lennard draws out the implications for that in arguing—
in his own form of ideology—that the chief responsibility
of therapists is to improve the quality of life of patients,
both inside the hospital, and eventually, for outside the
hospital. The goal of therapy today, and the institutional
arrangements of hospitals themselves, ought to aim toward that goal—as, of course, they often do not. What his
study of this particular mental institution shows is that its
ideological position is close to his own; that its institutional
arrangements do not lead to the kind of patients' suffering
that such arrangements often do, and are—on the contrary—instrumental in relieving some of the suffering. By
implication, Lennard's blunt reminder that much of mental illness is presently incurable brings those forms of illness into alignment with all the other, non-psychiatric,
chronic illnesses which finally are beginning to get the attention they merit as *the* contemporary form of illness;
needing new modes of treatment and management, both
medical and non-medical.

    While directing attention to one particular program,
the themes that emerge in *The Psychiatric Hospital* will be of
great interest to all those concerned with understanding
chronic mental illness, the organization of treatment process and the dynamics of change, whether they be clinicians or behavioral scientists.

Anselm Strauss, Ph.D.

FOREWORD

On my first contact with Henry Lennard 20 years ago I was impressed by his unusual combination of clinical and sociological concerns and had the thought that someday I would ask him to undertake a study of High Point Hospital. On my invitation, he spent some days with us in 1973. Together with a colleague he wrote a brief review of the hospital which I distributed to the profession.

At that time we made an attempt to bridge the gap between our disciplines. I recognized that we had much in common, and that he would eventually appreciate my thinking about hospital care. However, our relationship and exchange of views would need to be extensive. Our differences, as I saw them, became evident in his first report. First, there was his wariness of the proprietary hospital itself and of long term in-hospital treatment of the mentally ill. Very prominent were his objections against the use, and overuse, as he saw it, of medications. He also expressed reservations regarding the structuring of the treatment program, especially in relation to what he saw as its suppression of the patient's freedom and individuality. A principal point he made in his first report was that the hospital was too protective of the patient, and did not furnish him a sufficient "bridge" to the outside world.

Some 10 years elapsed before I sought Henry Lennard out again. He was cordial, and to my pleasant surprise indicated that he had thought about features of the High Point Hospital program in the intervening years as he had continued to study and compare mental institutions. He was therefore happy to accept my invitation to do a comprehensive and in-depth study of High Point Hospital. At the time we did not know that a book would be its issue. It was essentially to be a learning experience for both of us.

I have always been a socially oriented human being. Yet I recognized that as a physician and psychiatrist—no matter how socially oriented—in relation to the hospital I could not see the forest for the trees, if only because I was so heavily invested emotionally in the institution. The necessary expertise was his. I sensed that he had the necessary attribute of being nontraditional to do justice to this quite unorthodox institution. Thus High Point Hospital as a social structure was to be his field of study.

Ground rules laid out were brief and simple. He was to have free access to everyone, staff and patients alike, and freedom to say in writing whatever he believed. We both were to confer, speak freely, exchange our ideas and share our philosophies.

This book reflects the exchange of our ideas, and the

development of our relationship. Under his scrutiny I had opportunity to express and sharpen my ideas, and to hone new ideas which arose. My conscious effort was to affect his thinking, as I was sure his was to affect mine, with a plan that out of the experience some new ideas and approaches would evolve. A personal and professional relationship developed. I think we soon accepted that we would permit ourselves to be affected, one by the other. This could only come from an open recognition and sharing of our biases.

One aspect of our struggle related to the natural difference between the physician concerned with the individual and the researcher concerned with issues of social policy, the one bent on the eradication of pathology, and the other committed to acceptance of the disabled and societal modification so that the patient could live with the illness "with some quality of life." This was the fact, though each could see some of the other's chief thrust. Lennard, however, would have to appreciate my position that there was a fundamental disease process, not just a social disorder; that the doctor could do something about it; and that the ultimate goal was its eradication, with society's help. I would have to appreciate his view that cure is not tenable as a primary objective in work with the mentally ill and that the major treatment task was to help the ill person achieve a more satisfactory life, and for society to furnish him the opportunity for a more productive existence.

As our discussions continued they became more intimate, sometimes intense, provocative, and educational. At times our differences seemed a matter of semantics. At others, words carried different meanings for each of us. For instance, Lennard initially viewed "internalization" of the hospital's value system as the taking into one's self of the ideas of others, corresponding to superego development, an almost passive activity. For me "internalization" expressed an active process, namely, an individual's conscious selection, from an assortment of options, of a system of values to provide guidance. And this value system was subject to modification on the basis of continuing experience and maturation. While early experiences played a role, they were not necessarily foremost and did not necessarily limit one's options and choices. This view recognized the continuing reciprocal and changing relation between the individual and his environment.

We recognized that no matter how psychoanalytically oriented the hospital and how much it emphasized individual psychotherapy, what transpired in formal therapy settings was by no means the entire story of the therapeutic process. So obviously important was the hospital as a social structure that we could think of it as equally important to, if not more important than the psychotherapy itself. I often said to my medical staff that I could so disorganize the hospital milieu that their therapeutic sessions, no matter how often given, would be without effect.

As time went by I had to respond to questions of a rather personal nature with information necessary to the clinical sociologist: my early life experiences and the nature of the family in which I was raised; my early significant experiences and my early as well as current philosophy of life. I disclosed my basic belief in the social nature of man—that man's most precious possession was his humanity, and that this he owed to the presence of another human being. In the absence of another, man could have no humanity, and he therefore owed much to this other human being. If all beings could feel and believe this there would be no war, for everyone would be knowledgeably indebted to the other.

We agreed that the subject of values needed more detailed exploration and attention than it had received in studies of therapeutic milieus. We did know, however, that man did live by a value system. I believed that values arose out of man's interaction with others and their life experiences. Human beings developed value systems which could be quite different. The gratifying thing was that the culture could produce very positive values as well as very negative ones, and we had the facility to distinguish one from the other. It seemed to me that there was occurring a distinct polarization in values which was now dividing cultures and dividing the world. Out of this polarization a calamity might arise, or, more hopefully, a final healing and resolution. It might help if we knew what gave rise to the positive relational values. It did not seem helpful to believe that we were all instinctively evil. How then to account for the good?

I reviewed for Lennard the earliest stages of my education and training and experience in psychiatry, and what brought me to that field. I described the origins and stages of development of the hospital, and its earlier and current major problems. I had to review in some detail the task of bringing together the proper staff, both nonprofessional and professional, and then assist them in developing a philosophy that reinforces the core therapeutic approach. I had to permit him to view me in action so that he could understand the hospital's operating problems and how I solve them. Firsthand he could see the process of implementing the hospital's basic therapeutic approach.

It seemed necessary to air my apprehension about the future of psychiatry. In the light of the deinstitutionalization movement I detailed my dread and strong opposition to it. We discussed the prospects for hospital psychiatry, particularly the vitally important extended type so needed by many patients. I expressed my reservations about the theory of the "unconscious." While it might have been of help to us earlier this theory might now be hindering our progress and limiting our ability to do more clinically. Some brave new theory was needed to suit our innovative and creative therapeutic techniques. While we knew much we did not know essentially more than we did some 50 years ago. There was very much more to know than we already knew.

This discussion of the "unconscious" led to fruitful dialogue about the origins of consciousness, memory, and the process of recall. In some detail we discussed the ongoing and reciprocal relationship between man and his environment peopled by others. It was this experience that gave rise to consciousness, and recall was a new consciousness of an event that was created by continuing current experience. This experience, with the conscious participation of the person, created anew the memory of the earlier event, and thus the "memory." This approach did not require the construct, or theory, of the "unconscious," particularly as an operating and ongoing force.

As time went by it was gratifying to witness Lennard's increasing enthusiasm about High Point Hospital as a therapeutic context, and about the contribution that the book he was by this time writing would make to an understanding of therapeutic process. This naturally followed as he studied our clinical practice, observed the everyday life of the hospital, and saw good results with patients. He identified features of the program that illustrated social theories of change processes. I recall his satisfaction at explaining the concept of deuterolearning when he discovered its relation to the therapeutic process at High Point Hospital. I, of course, was excited about what was newfound knowledge for me and yet another facet of this complex therapeutic structure.

One aspect of the program remained a source of concern. Lennard found the staff of High Point Hospital devoted and dedicated. However, he found that they did not always seem to show sufficient comprehension of my basic therapeutic thesis. He would have preferred that they had. I could only respond that, if he were right, this was an inevitable facet of a therapeutic structure that required constant attention. Again, it would not be different from the gap in the grasp of rationality that existed between the psychiatrist and patient. That, too, required constant work.

I founded High Point Hospital in 1951. I have learned much now from its exposure to the scrutiny of an able sociologist. Therapeutic aspects of it have been identified and described in this book which otherwise would have continued unknown. Awareness of these should advance psychiatric hospital practice and evolve a more constructive and useful theoretical substructure for it. The study has been a rewarding experience for me, and I am sure for Henry Lennard likewise. I know he joins me in the hope that this book will be equally exciting and stimulating for its readers.

We had agreed that Lennard would have full freedom to study all aspects of the hospital's life. However, there are some observations reported which in my opinion as a psychiatrist may be seen differently. Some recommendations are made which I believe would not necessarily add to the program's therapeutic value. It would be too much to expect that two persons with such diverse backgrounds and convictions should come to complete agreement. I would point to two examples. Lennard sees the prescription of medication for the "convenience" of personnel, whereas I see such medication as a necessary calming of the patient for his own welfare as well as the general social well-being. He sees "restriction" of the patient as sometimes unnecessary limitation of the patient's "freedom." I see such "restriction" as vital limitation because the patient cannot as yet rationally use his freedom. It is not much different from the limitation we place on the patient with a fracture until he heals sufficiently to bear weight. We limit the psychiatric patient until he is sufficiently well to bear greater responsibility. With regard to other examples I leave to the reader what is always his responsibility, namely to read with an inquiring mind as he goes along.

Alexander Gralnick, M.D.

Part I

A CONCEPTUAL FRAMEWORK

Chapter 1

SOCIAL THERAPY:
A COMPREHENSIVE MODEL

In this book I will describe—in some respects more comprehensively than has been done so far—the essential elements of social healing processes: the social context and processes that effect changes in the social behavior, values, and symptoms of schizophrenic persons. While the sources of the theory are many, it will be illustrated here primarily through reference to one treatment program that I have come to know extremely well. It is a program that has, since its inception, struggled to proceed on the assumption that it is possible to design a social and physical context, with a particular expectational and value structure, that brings about not only behavioral change but also modifies symptomatology and lifelong vulnerability to psychiatric disorder.

In group and family therapies and social and community psychiatry, the operative focus of most professional activities has too often revolved around attempts to change the behavior of individuals and to effect change by the manipulation of the psychological rather than to change interactional patterns and the social context. Therapeutic milieus are often places in which therapy is done to individuals, rather than contexts that are in themselves therapeutic; and the thrust of community mental health programs has been, more often than not, to make individual treatment or consultation available, rather than to create social contexts that are therapeutic.

Therapeutic effects are achieved only partially through direct relations between staff and patients. The hospital environment as a whole plays a more important role than any specific form of staff-patient contact or therapeutic modality. Thus it becomes critical to look at the context as a whole as the appropriate focus for what is therapeutic.

While many elements required for change contexts are also present in other psychiatric and rehabilitative programs studied by others and myself,[1-4] an extensive analysis and study of the High Point Hospital program enables me to identify and describe in detail the variety of contextual and social process features requisite and conducive to patient change.

Most of the patients who participate in the High Point program are young—under twenty years of age—and have a diagnosis of schizophrenia or schizoaffective disorder. While the value of such diagnoses are limited for disorders that have rather "nebulous boundaries," there are distinct features. The majority of patients, adolescents and young adults, have grown up in social contexts where noxious transactions predominate, and have become severely disabled; and most exhibit symptoms associated with a diagnosis of schizophrenia.

If the diagnosis and treatment of mental disorder were an exact science, as few branches of medicine and behavioral science are, one would expect that a specific diagnosis would result in a specific treatment, notwithstanding where and by whom it was administered. This is not the case! The form of psychiatric treatment administered is more often contingent on which hospital system, facility, or program a patient happens to get to, and on what treatment modalities happen to be fashionable at a particular time and place.

The clinician and researcher would at the very least wish to be able to specify which treatment context and modality is the most appropriate for particular kinds of persons, and to describe, in detail, the social and therapeutic processes through which a beneficial healing influence is to be achieved.

It is the objective of this book to identify and describe such characteristics of a therapeutic social context—the social processes, communicational parameters, attitudes and expectations—that by themselves, or acting synergistically, produce change. I will present the mosaic of such elements essential for the program's instructions to be "metabolized" and learned; i.e., for patients to adopt the role behaviors, rules of conduct, and value orientations expected and considered functional.

Yet in stating this objective of our study I am aware of Joe Zubin's observation[5] reached after a lifetime of study of schizophrenic persons, regarding the "abysmal" ignorance that surrounds the schizophrenic disorder, ". . . lack of a precise definition of schizophrenia, . . . ignorance of etiology, . . . lack of knowledge regarding when and how to intervene . . . what the goals of intervention should be . . ."

But if we believe with Zubin that, at this time, the most useful position is one that views schizophrenia as a product of an enduring vulnerability and the effects of external stressors that exceed the threshold of tolerance, then it becomes necessary to focus on the characteristics of an interactional environment that raises that threshold.[6]

The description of such interactional features and processes essential to change offered here has been made possible by the application of sociological concepts such as micro-order, situational adjustment, forms of therapeutic work, and deutero-role learning. I have also explored the usefulness of a variety of formulations in thinking about context and change, such as "appropriate dosage of social interventions;" "ideas as viruses;" and "schizophrenia as a cultural value system." Special emphasis is also given to the role played by the physical setting in facilitating a therapeutic program.

For the change model set forth here it is not, however, necessary to be committed to a particular conception of schizophrenia or its etiology as an illness, or alternatively as an "aggregate of formal characteristics of personal interaction" (Bateson),[7] as a "*Lebensform*" (Wittgenstein),[8] or " . . . as a specific state of personality with its own way of living" (Fromm-Reichmann).[9]

The social process model set forth in this book encompasses all of the above conceptions, since the goals of treatment and social intervention are essentially similar, irrespective of one's position on etiology or the nature of the schizophrenic person.

Participation in any system of treatment and social intervention should enable persons to "live with" their illness, disability, or different mode of being. At the very least, change should reduce distressing symptoms, enable schizophrenic persons to relate to other human beings with competence and pleasure, enable such persons "to find for themselves, without injury to their neighbors their own sources of satisfaction and security,"[10] and reduce the rejection and contempt with which schizophrenic persons are treated.

I will specify the range of social processes that make possible the learning of instrumental skills, social-relational values and the enhancement of self-esteem and personhood.

Among the significant social processes and programmatic features that will be described in the book are the following:

The placement and movement of patients through groups with distinctive responsibilities and privileges, and subject to slowly increasing social expectations and pressures;

An expanded conception of therapeutic work that includes the therapists' participation in all facets of the work of hospitals, and requires role behaviors not ordinarily associated with traditional hospital role structures, such as Attentional, Informational, Competence, and Trust work;

Attention to role induction, role learning, and resocialization processes, and to providing conditions favorable to deuterolearning;

The utilization of the physical-architectural features of the hospital as a therapeutic modality and as reinforcement of program objectives;

A conception of the therapeutic program as a value learning context. The set of relational values to be learned are made explicit and communicated;

Monitoring of the operation of the system as a whole and rapid response to expectational or communicational disequilibria;

An evolving theory of effective dosage of therapeutic interventions that specifies timing and duration of exposure to treatment required for change.

Some of the features of the High Point program described here are also characteristic of other psychiatric and rehabilitation programs. I suggest, however, that all of these elements need to be present for a program to be an effective agent for social healing processes to occur.

While "for some it is bad news to think that interpersonal relationships, family systems, and society itself may be a major determinant of the disorder,"[11] it is good news indeed that social contexts can be devised and maintained that reverse the course of the disorder, or at the least ameliorate the secondary iatrogenesis that can be brought about by an unfortunate human environment.

To understand one treatment context that illustrates the variety of process characteristics required to meet this goal is a contribution to our understanding of the dynamics of healing and change.

Yet we must also be reminded that the rehabilitation, integration, and well-being of schizophrenic persons is not only contingent upon treatment contexts, but is also influenced by the perception and treatment of such persons by members of their community prior and subsequent to hospitalization.

The Psychiatric Hospital makes explicit how social contexts modify and change human behavior. This book examines the extent to which behavior, including psychological impairment, psychiatric symptomatology, and deviant behavior generally are subject to change within social contexts.

Current psychiatric formulations about milieu or therapeutic community treatments do not do justice to interactional process properties and system characteristics of "therapeutic" social contexts. Discussion too often is limited to a description of static variables (containment, structure, support, etc.) rather than concerned with dynamic and intrinsic properties of the contexts themselves.

I view differences in social contexts as a function of what transpires within them interactionally. From this point of view a social context consists of configurations and sequences of interaction, particular thematic emphases, and attitudinal orientations to these interactions and emphases. Social contexts represent special interactional and expectational environments. Social healing contexts exhibit very specific interactional process characteristics and related role and value orientations. They also require a physical setting that actively reinforces their special interactional role and value character.

Chapter 2

THE THERAPEUTIC COMMUNITY
IN THEORY AND ACTION

If one asks mental health professionals what it is they do, the response will most often be, "I do therapy." This assumes that whatever transpires during a treatment setting, in individual or group therapy, or in a psychiatric institution is, by definition, "therapeutic." This attitude is so much a part of the professional ethos that it obscures the fact that programs and interventions undertaken for the purpose of effecting therapeutic change may sometimes, despite the best intentions, be counterproductive. On the other hand, dramatic therapeutic changes can and do occur in persons participating in some social institutions. It therefore becomes important to learn what kind of therapeutic arrangements bring about such beneficial changes in their members, and to identify those parameters and processes most likely responsible.

"Therapeutic community" has come to be an accepted term for a treatment environment and therapeutic program that goes well beyond the doctor-patient relationship of "individual psychotherapy." Since the early work of the British psychiatrist, Maxwell Jones[1] in the late 1940s, hospital care and, more recently, community care centers, have moved steadily in the direction of using the structure and process of the program itself as a principal theapeutic "instrument."

The therapeutic community represents to some a specific treatment method "as specific as psychoanalysis or somatic therapy." When it is working at its best, it is comprised of many different therapeutic inputs. It is a social structure designed to be the primary instrument in the helping process, where all interactions and relationships are relevant and potentially therapeutic. The staff members must strive for the condition where they are able to prize the importance of their own contribution and respect and value the contribution of their colleagues, regardless of their hierarchical position "Because of the powerful psychological impact this organized social system can make on the patient, it is essential that values, the cultural attitudes of the community, be continually identified, examined and modified."[2]

For some, the term "therapeutic milieu" has come to mean a system of organizing relationships in such a way that patients share in both the management of their lives and their plans of treatment. Many such programs play down the role of the staff as therapists, maintaining that everyone is a therapist for everyone else. "Therapeutic community" in these programs designates procedures which are typically "democratic" as opposed to "authoritarian;" treatment-oriented as contrasted with custodial-oriented; humanitarian instead of oppressive; and flexible as opposed to rigid. This conception, however, only considers limited aspects of the therapeutic context.

In this chapter I will outline a framework for assessing therapeutic contexts generally; that is, specify the dimensions, processes, and problems that need to be included in the examination of any program. If these can be defined, the range of choices available to any program becomes clearer, and potential contradictions attain greater legibility.

ROLE CONCEPTIONS

Decisions around the division of labor in a psychiatric program go far beyond the specifications of duties and functions. We include the expectations persons have of each other and of themselves for performing their roles in the total process. The ways in which roles are defined is strategic. The meaning and enactment of the roles labeled as doctor, nurse, attendant, and patient provide definition and boundaries for the behavior of the participants. A clearly defined set of roles according to graded authority may be seen from one point of view as promoting distance between patients and staff and among staff, but from another perspective it promotes a highly legible environment with the reduction of anxiety around questions of who one is and how one is to behave in the setting.

On the other hand, "role diffusion" allows staff to interact with patients and each other along a wider array of issues. Role diffusion in some therapeutic communities even implies that "decision making as well as leadership responsibilities are assigned not merely on the basis of one's staff position."

The concept of "role diffusion," as used by Hoffman and others,[3] however, does not do justice to the complex requirements for staff "work" in a genuinely therapeutic system. It has become clear that the conception of the everyday role performances of professional and nonprofessional staff in such contexts must be differentiated from how roles are enacted in traditional hospital and institutional settings. In a therapeutic context such as High Point Hospital, as we shall explore in detail in this book, the everyday work and conception of therapeutic work[4]—of the staff as a whole—encompasses a range of activities and concerns not ordinarily associated with the traditional role functions of physician, nurse, social worker, and so forth. Yet it is appropriate to describe these forms of staff functioning as work since they exhibit all the characteristics of work; they involve expenditures of energy, time, and skill, and can be both described and taught.

Therapeutic Work

Professional staff members participate in the work of seven patient committees that are concerned with a variety of patient activities and the everyday operations of the hospital. In addition to their work on committees, professionals are expected to participate in activities that we have described as comprising forms of therapeutic work such as:

Attentional Work—to pay attention to the small, mundane occurrences of everyday patient life in the hospital, and to be alert to all aspects of the social and physical enviroment;

Informational Work—to obtain and transmit information, not only information required for clinical work, but also that concerning everyday occurrences in the life of the hospital;

Membership Work—to sacrifice some part of professional self-image, and renounce some measure of professional autonomy in order to function as a member of a multidisciplinary treatment team;

Trust Work—to build trust in staff and program and to investigate and resolve inconsistencies and discrepancies in treatment policies and commitments made to patients;

Competence Work—to assist patients directly to enhance their social, interactional, and instrumental competencies.

RESOCIALIZATION PROCESSES

How social contexts bring about changes in patterns of behavior is one aspect of a larger problem that has consistently concerned social scientists; how "social behavior moves (or fails to move) people to act in ways other people want them to act."[5]

Socialization has emerged as the single concept to encompass the processes involved. The term social control has also been invoked to describe this range of phenomena. The concept of "social control," however, has for some a perjorative connotation. It has been equated with efforts by social groups, especially those with power, to manage and constrain non-conformists or persons vulnerable due to their lack of power or access to resources. However, the sociologist Goode suggests that the term social control be used in its broadest sense, that is, to "refer to all aspects of control by anyone in relation to anyone . . ."[6]

The Goode Hypotheses

A set of hypotheses suggested by Goode permit us to understand just how change in attitudes and behavior comes about, whether in a family setting or in a therapeutic community setting; and how the processes of learning norms and rules of interpersonal conduct can be facilitated.

These hypotheses are congruent with much that I have observed in the day-to-day operations of therapeutic communities, and is especially germane to the findings of the study of the High Point Hospital program. The first hypothesis, one that has been accepted widely across the behavioral sciences, is that "people's behavior is shaped or affected by the esteem (approbation) that others give to them or withdraw from them . . ."

Goode adds the proposition that human beings "have been socialized to need this deference or esteem, and these responses become ends in themselves. . ." From "the earliest period of childhood socialization approval is accompanied by love and affection, and disapproval by anger, rejection, and sometimes physical hurt. . . If others do not recognize our worth, we are dismayed, annoyed or bitter."[7]

It is important to realize that in socialization and social exchange processes "people are more than likely to take on a task or duty that they had no great wish to assume . . . The theory of cognitive dissonance is relevant here as well, in that it asserts that persons' behaviors and especially their attitudes are more likely to be shaped if they are faced with contrary alternatives between difficult choices and are somewhat gently, but successfully, pressed to follow one" (of these alternatives).[8]

To take on a different set of values and moral commitments, to behave in new and functional ways, is enhanced by "raised inducement rather than by physical punishment, by social rejection or threat of withdrawing love or respect rather than by deprivation of material things, by close physical or emotional contact. . . rather than by severe threats at a distance, persuasion rather than by physical barriers, by permitting temptation and giving trust . . . rather than removing entirely what is forbidden."[9]

The interactional structure of the High Point program incorporates each of the social learning principles outlined here. At High Point tasks are graded in terms of difficulty, so that patients may initially achieve success in minor behavioral improvements. These changes are noted and praise is given. For more global changes in values and behavior patients are given increasing respect and esteem. This is further validated by a system of graded privileges in the life of the community that are made explicit and known by all patients. Threats are avoided and explanation and persuasion are utilized with close attention to the dysfunctional behaviors involved. Staff provide models of trustworthy behavior, and patients are given increasing levels of trust for their conduct, relations, and responsibility for each other. Even if trust is violated, consequences, though explicit, are limited in duration. Patients may fail to live up to expectations, and yet expectations will be maintained that sooner or later congruent and appropriate behavior will be achieved.

SITUATIONAL ADJUSTMENT

Those convinced of the effectiveness of therapeutic context to bring about change must question the assumption that human beings are essentially unchanging. In the concept of situational adjustment the sociologist Becker summarizes the growing evidence that persons, moving into a new context, will, given certain conditions, learn the requirements for functioning within that social context. To the extent that persons develop a desire to continue in the situation, they can deliver the required performances and turn themselves into the kind of person the situation demands. Becker has theorized about the mechanisms whereby participation in social organizations produces change. "The person, as he participates in social interaction, constantly takes the role of others, viewing what he does and is about to do from their viewpoint, imputing to his own actions the meanings he anticipates others will impute to them. . . . One important implication of this view is that people are not free to act as their own inner dispositions (however we may conceptualize them) dictate. . . . Instead, they act as they are constrained by the actions of their co-participants."[10] Becker explains that resocialization involves many "sequences of smaller and more numerous situational adjustments. . . sequences and combinations of small units of adjustment produce the larger units of role learning."[11]

Within the High Point Hospital program patients make situational adjustments within ever increasing orbits and time frames. In the course of the patient's career in the hospital they participate in a series of social contexts, each more difficult than the preceding ones. As they move through each, they test and strengthen their social skills, and acquire changing appraisals of themselves, of others, and of themselves in relation to others. Bettelheim, who fashioned an effective psychiatric inpatient program in some respects similar to that of High Point, asserts that "higher coping can only be achieved under the impact of challenges which are graded, so that each level can be mastered with just a minimum of further effort . . . a good mental institution has to help the patient, small step by small step, learn to cope."[12]

Among the conditions necessary for changes in attitudes, behavior, and associated "coping skills" is at least minimal motivation to continue participation in the context—a desire to continue to interact, to communicate, and to be connected with other persons located within one's context. The principle mechanism by which this is accomplished appears to be through the building up of attachments to such other persons—that is, by emotional communication with them, so that the individual is sensitized to their attitudes. To the extent, then, that patients acquire such attachments and motivation, however rudimentary, to interact, they are subject to resocialization and change by a genuinely therapeutic environment. Human beings, no matter how psychologically disturbed, require and depend on some contact with other human beings.

Chapter 3

NORMATIVE STRUCTURE

A therapeutic context creates an interruption of basic patterns. It changes the significant norms, activities, and the everyday context that has made up the patient's previous life. It seeks to embed the person in a new social network and place him or her in a field in which the strongest influences pull for involvement in activities other than the behavior which has come to be recognized as his or her "symptoms."

ORGANIZATION OF TREATMENT CONTEXT

Within that new context certain specific conditions must be fulfilled if that context is to be therapeutic. These have to do with the norms governing daily interaction, the learning and practice of new role behaviors, and the manner in which participation in the context itself becomes an agent for the process of change (deuterolearning).

The first feature of any therapeutic effort to bring about change is to move the individual into a context whose modes of operation are distinctly different from the social groups he has just left. The norms governing the behavior of all members of the treatment program must serve the purpose of the organization. At least some norms of the treatment organization will be the opposite of those held by previous groups to which the members belonged.

Social Control

A degree of social control is exercised over all patients in the treatment setting. Positive and negative sanctions are strong and visible. Among these are procedures for progress in the program, and channels for the expression of interpersonal approval and disapproval. Such social control mechanisms maintain the hospital's purpose and strengthen the commitment of individual members to the program.

All members of the organization, staff and patients alike, must be able to represent the program's normative system, both through an understanding and honoring of its norms, and by exercising sanctions. This function should also not be the exclusive prerogative of "staff." The presence of social controls must in turn be matched by the opportunity for personal gratification and growth among the members who abide by the prevailing norms. A sense of community and identification, pride in the effectiveness of the hospital, and options for increased involvement in the activities of the program, are among these gratifications.

Procedures for Change

Progress through the different phases of the therapeutic program should be based on universalistic criteria. Every patient entering the hospital must share a clear conception of the stages and levels of the program. Movement within the system should proceed through a sequence of formally defined stages, with appropriate rituals marking the passage from one stage to another.

The staff and patients at High Point clearly share a set of norms which govern their behavior at the hospital. The hospital attempts to establish a consensus between staff and patient on what has led persons to become ill and disabled and how they can improve and become able to function. Many of these norms are in direct opposition to those held by new patients and by social groups to which they previously belonged. For example, High Point staff oppose the idea that each individual is the best judge of what he should or shouldn't do, and stress an emphasis on mutual consideration and trust.

The formation of subgroups opposed or disloyal to the hospital is strongly discouraged. Graded levels of authority and responsibility decrease the formation of coalitions among subgroups. Positive and negative sanctions governing both staff and patients are strong and visible. Procedures for changing status in the hospital are familiar and clear. These mechanisms maintain the hospital's purpose and serve to strengthen the commitment of individual participants to the treatment program.

Staff and patients are expected to act as agents for the hospital's normative system. This function is not the exclusive prerogative of the staff or of only certain patients. All participants in this community relate to one another in some respects as members of a large extended family, even while the rights and obligations among the membership are not equally distributed. All are expected to uphold the hospital's standards and its rules. Staff and patients are not pitted against one another as they are in many hospitals.

Role Definition

The presence of social controls is matched by the clarity of role instructions, particularly surrounding the opportunities for progress in the system. Patients know in simple terms what they must do to move from one group to the next and what behaviors mark their progression. They also know what rights accrue to which patients at what level. The ambiguity of the environment has been reduced to a minimum in those areas relating to what patient behaviors produce what effects or lead to rewards or rejections. The consensus that respect for the prevailing norms will be recognized and rewarded leads to a sense of community and a pride in the effectiveness of the hospital.

At the same time too, new staff members, professionals and nonprofessionals alike, are part of a normative induction process. Here too expectations are clearly expressed and repeated. Learning a philosophy of the "hospital as a therapeutic instrument" and how such a philosophy can be implemented through the day-to-day work of the staff is anticipated to take time. However, staff who fail to learn the normative system may find themselves in a continuous struggle with their colleagues and may ultimately choose to leave the system.

In participating in a therapeutic context, patients learn that in that particular social setting there are certain behaviors, expectations, and sequences of events that are appropriate and certain others that are not. Induction into the therapeutic system occurs through receipt of explicit role instructions and through the inferences drawn from this role teaching.

Such role learning has the broadest of applications and is in itself "therapeutic." The contextual structure of a therapeutic environment represents a highly characteristic pattern of interaction and norms to which a patient is repeatedly exposed, and ultimately limits and shapes the patient's behavior. Participation in such an interaction context characteristically encourages a patient to deepen and accelerate his or her further involvement. The successful experience of interaction in the High Point Hospital environment is a message to the patient: "You (the patient) are

competent (or soon shall be) and have the ability to function interactionally and you are a valued human being."

The staff become "experts in living" and take the responsibility for communicating about the roles and requirements of the context in which the patients now find
themselves and within which they will remain as long as
they are in treatment.

Because successful participation in social situations requires complementarity of expectations and behavior,
problems develop when the level of role system information provided in the course of interaction falls below the
level required for appropriate functioning. Untoward outcomes for the system and its members result when role
prescriptions and instructions are poorly conveyed and
are ambiguous.

During the early stages of involvement in a new setting, a considerable amount of interaction is devoted to
role instructions and clarification of how the patient is to
relate to what is now happening to and around him.

A minimum amount of socialization is required to
generate and maintain any social system. A failure to provide such minimal levels of socialization in the course of
the interaction with new patients is responsible for the failure of programs to achieve their goals. A therapeutic context is responsible for achieving dual objectives. Within,
members are to be socialized to function as part of the
treatment setting; but they must be taught ultimately how
to function in other social contexts as well. Both of these
objectives can be accomplished successfully as long as the
two tasks remain complementary. They fail when one objective competes or conflicts with the other. Hence, when
relations among staff take the form of mystification, not
only will the primary task of role induction fail, but the entire setting loses its credibility and effectiveness to perform
the goal of teaching the membership how to behave adequately in other social contexts.

Deuterolearning

Deuterolearning is a concept we owe to Gregory Bateson,[1] and refers to second-order learning, or learning how to learn. In learning a language, for example, one learns not only the language but also about how to proceed in the learning of the language, that is, to become alert to the position of nouns and verbs, appropriate tenses, and so forth.

I have previously suggested that the concept of deuterolearning was useful to an understanding of the psychotherapy interaction, that at its best encourages the process of deuterolearning.[2] The question now became to identify how and in which aspects a complex therapeutic context such as High Point Hospital facilitates the process of deuterolearning, or the acquisition of skills to learn the requirements for functioning within a variety of social contexts and systems.

The continuous monitoring and attention to the micro-order of everyday interaction processes by persons skilled in observing functional and dysfunctional interaction—a form of therapeutic work especially characteristic of the High Point program—emerges as the principle mechanism that facilitated the process of deuterolearning in patients.

Value Learning

Whether or not it is admitted or denied, explicit or implicit, participation in a social system involves the communication of values. Participants act and expect others to act in accordance with specific rules, principles, and priorities. Just as it is not feasible *not* to communicate, so it is not possible *not* to express values.

Some therapists are explicit about their value system,

and conceive it to be part of therapeutic work: to assist patients to acquire and to live by principles described as "healthier" or "more functional."

While some analysts may deny explicit value education as a goal of treatment, there is evidence that judgments of therapeutic success or failure by therapists are often related to the extent to which patients have adopted value systems congruent with theirs.

Fromm-Reichmann argues that "It is not correct to say that there is *no* inherent set of values concerned with the goals of psychotherapy. . . . The psychiatrist should not be afraid of being aware of these standards (values) or to admit that these are the basic standards which guide him in his therapeutic dealings with patients, no matter how eager he may be to establish his personal evaluational neutrality."[3]

The problem of values becomes even more complex when we consider a therapeutic program in a psychiatric facility—with patients participating over a period of months or longer—in which they interact with a variety of personnel and with other patients. Each day patients adapt to a myriad of expectations, instructions, and institutional rules, and engage in a range of social transactions that are scrutinized and commented on in detail.

As High Point's program evolved over the years, an explicit concern with patients' value system has become a priority of the therapeutic work of High Point Hospital treatment system.

High Point's program is based on a set of related assumptions: (a) that staff be clear about the sets of values governing the relations among staff, and of staff with patients; (b) that it is part of therapeutic "work" for all treatment personnel to be an agent, spokesperson, and representative of the therapeutic community's value system; (c) moreover, that it is a part of therapeutic "work" to assist patients in the examination of their values; and (d) that the program must represent a social context conducive to the learning and adoption of values for a "constructive," "less painful," and "healthier" life.

Relational Ethics

In its concern with value issues the High Point Hospital program occupies a rather unique position among psychiatric institutions. The values communicated by staff, and the extent of their adoption by patients become a focus of attention in the study. Values that receive higher priority at High Point than elsewhere may be described by Boszormenyi-Nagy's term "relational ethics." Ethical theories traditionally focus on the individual, and stress the autonomy, "rights," dignity, and freedom of individual persons. At High Point there is an additional emphasis on an ethic of mutual consideration, on relational fairness, and on merited trust. In relational ethics as developed in theory by Ivan Nagy and practiced at High Point, there is an emphasis on the "simultaneous multilateral consideration of more than one human being." To merit trust, to treat others fairly and be treated fairly by them, to assist and be assisted by others are values that are given high priority in the program.

Values and Schizophrenia

Implicit in the program is the assumption that value priorities and change in values may be central to an understanding of the life experiences of schizophrenic persons, and that a value change—literally the adoption of a different cultural value system—may be connected to the amelioration of symptoms and being able to live with the schizophrenic vulnerability.

The social world of schizophrenic persons is organized around such value dimensions as trust-mistrust, approach-withdrawal, justice-injustice, hope-despair, and so on.

The shared preoccupation with these values may be viewed both as a symptom and as a coping mechanism (analogous to how symptoms of physical disorder are both an expression of the disease, as well as a form of coping with the disease).

To the extent that patients live in a social context that emphasizes such relational values as trust and trustworthiness, fairness, justice, and mutual consideration, and adopt these in organizing their behavior and expectations, symptoms diminish. High Point's emphasis on relational values is not at the expense of depreciating the patient's dignity and personhood. Nonetheless, balancing an emphasis on relational and individual focussed values within the framework of an inpatient hospital program leads to "value dilemmas" and that will be made explicit in this book.

COMMUNICATION AND VULNERABILITY

Patterns of human interaction vary in both quantitative and qualitative characteristics and may therefore generate difficulties for individuals along either continuum. Certain qualitative contents of communication are easier to cope with than others. Positive and supporting communications create less stress than negative and demeaning ones. But of equal importance in determining the difficulties an individual will have in interacting with a given treatment milieu is the quantity of such noxious communications and their distribution over time.

When therapeutic efforts occur within a "difficult" communicational field they may "get nowhere" and produce a sense of frustration and dissatisfaction on the part of staff. Not only do the communicational contexts that envelop patients vary in difficulty, the patients themselves differ in their ability to adapt and to deal with the immediate environment. Some patients are more vulnerable to destructive communications, and less capable of meeting excessive demands. Such vulnerability can be due to differential thresholds for the perception of attacks or demands or to an inability to neutralize them.

Sullivan firmly believed that schizophrenic persons "surrounded by affection and intimacy rather than hate or humiliation are better able to reorganize their personalities." He cautioned—an admonition particularly relevant at this time—that "patients showing improvement under such treatment should not be hurried out of the therapeutic environment into unfavorable situations that might cause them to have relapses."[4]

The Neutralizing Capabilities

Psychological vulnerability may be conceived of as analogous to an organism's ability to process and neutralize noxious substances to which it has been exposed. Just as organisms can neutralize only small amounts of poisons encountered at infrequent intervals, so some persons are able to meet demands only when these demands are received in small doses, well-spaced in time. Therapeutic environments cease to be such when the level of difficulty they present or the demands inherent in interacting within them exceed the neutralizing or coping abilities of the patients they serve.

If, indeed, variations in contextual difficulties are crucial, then attention must be directed to the interactional and expectational characteristics of therapeutic environments. The social context of the patients' everyday life must be so organized that communicational acts and expectations do not exceed their tolerance thresholds and do not tax patients beyond their ability to neutralize frustrating and discordant communication. Sometimes neuroleptic drugs are used to achieve this objective. One effect of these drugs is to increase thresholds for processing demands and noxious stimuli. Unfortunately, however, their use may at the same time reduce the pressure toward the creation of circumstances more suitable to the everyday human needs of the patients.

Therapeutic environments may be static or repetitive or they may be dynamic and progressive. Repetitive interactions, in the popular idiom, "do not go anywhere." Neither the relationship between the participants nor the interactional process seems to evolve. Such therapy systems do not exhibit expected phases of growth and differentiation.

Settings in which there is no interactional development or evolution may be deemed harmful, while those that provide the experience of participating in an evolving relationship or interactive process may be deemed beneficial or therapeutic. The development and programming of interaction requires the collaboration of every member of the therapeutic community. A competent parent helps a child to move through difficult interactive phases and a skilled therapeutic team does much the same thing for patients.

SIGNIFICANCE OF PHYSICAL SETTING

While it is understood that the physical architectural features within which a therapeutic program is located are important, their specific role and therapeutic potential have generally not been made explicit.

Bettelheim, who more than most clinicians has been sensitive to the role of hospital architecture in the treatment process writes that "at present . . . there are no definite and successful models for designing physical structure (and internal organization) of a mental institution."[5]

The physical setting in which treatment occurs influences behavior, social interaction, and self-esteem. In addition to the purely functional overt aspects, every building also conveys a range of "covert" messages. The physical setting of a therapeutic program represents a powerful form of metacommunication regarding the programs conception of the patient, and instructions as to how patients are to experience themselves, to relate to others, and to remain the same or to change.

The physical setting and features of High Point Hospital have, over the years, become a significant element and reinforcer of its program.

Subjecting High Point's environment to the detailed analysis presented in this study serves two objectives: to make explicit and analyze the use of the physical-architectural environment in meeting the objectives of a particular program; and to utilize the knowledge gained from such an analysis to suggest how specific environmental arrangements can provide support for the therapeutic and rehabilitative goals of psychiatric facilities generally.

For example, at High Point rules governing restriction of movement in the building are used in conjunction with territorial rewards permitting access to and use of particular attractive spaces. These rules and rewards reflect a balance that is maintained between protecting patients from doing damage to themselves and others, and trusting the patient to share some of the responsibility for self and others.

The environmental progress that patients made during their stay at a psychiatric hospital, from being initially rather restricted in freedom of movement, to gaining an increasing measure of freedom to use building and grounds, thus parallels the patient's growing sense of responsibility, self control, and sense of self worth.

DOSAGE OF SOCIAL THERAPIES

Most physical treatment modalities are based on theories of dosage. Such theories include assumptions regarding the appropriate dose of the treatment modality (e.g., drug, radiation exposure, etc.) administered, the frequency of administration, and the nature of the biological mechanisms involved.

However, there does not exist any comparable and validated theory of dosage for social system interventions, for psychotherapy or for the forms of social therapy described in this book.

Yet these forms of intervention are based on implicit conceptions of "dosage" and duration of treatment. I will make explicit assumptions as to the "dose" and duration of "application" that optimize the effects of therapeutic contexts such as High Point Hospital. I am concerned with the variety of social therapy interventions that result in enduring changes in behavior and in social relationships, that result in an increase in patients' understanding of the principles that regulate their functioning in everyday life situations, and with their ability to utilize such principles in different settings.

The High Point Hospital program has been accumulating information, over the past 3 decades, that helps define the parameters of a theory of "dosage" for the effects of therapeutic social systems. It has been found[6] that the program's favorable effects can best be observed and documented in patients who have been participating in the program for the duration of a year or longer.

I will describe the social therapy equivalent of a treatment dose; that is, the elements, patterns, and processes to which patients must be exposed, and the types of repeated, progressively difficult, and synergistic experiences required for a "therapeutic context," such as High Point Hospital, to bring about change.

Part II

METHODOLOGY

Chapter 4

METHODS AND ISSUES

INTRODUCTION

I have been familiar with the work of High Point Hospital since the early 1960s. In 1972 a colleague and I made a number of field visits to High Point Hospital to describe the structure and process of its treatment program.[1] In the light of further experience with the study of a number of therapeutic communities,[2,3] a more extensive study of High Point's program was begun in the fall of 1982. The current study then represents a part of a program of research and analysis of therapeutic contexts designed to effect change.

High Point Hospital's program proceeds from the premise that a well-staffed, thoughtfully designed institution can provide a healing context for individuals who have become disturbed through their associations in their world. The program has a dual commitment, to both a medical and a social model of psychic distress. While on the one hand patients are seen as "sick" and in need of treatment from medical staff, they are also seen as having come to their "illness" through participating in noxious human relationships, and from having to meet demands which exceeded their coping skills.

The idea that High Point Hospital represents a therapeutic context to which patients are exposed gradually replaced a description of the hospital as a place where psychotherapy is performed with patients needing hospitalization. While the individual psychiatrist-patient relationship is still viewed as an important ingredient in the total treatment plan, what is significant about this change is that the key process in restoring the patient to functioning is now seen as social learning in the sense of socialization and resocialization.

While the conclusions of the earlier study were reinforced in this more extensive effort, additional insights into some unique features of High Point's program emerged as well. Some of these have significant implications for programs designed to change persons, and especially for the work of inpatient settings with schizophrenic persons and others severely mentally disabled.

THE PROBLEM OF DESCRIPTION

Studies of treatment settings employ a variety of research methods: clinical descriptions, interviews and questionnaires, rating scales, objective and participant observation, analysis of patient records and of demographic data on patient and staff characteristics, and of data on organizational attributes of the hospital or treatment facility.

In the past studies I have worked with a combination of these methods, and been especially committed to the development of quantitative methods for the analysis of ongoing behavior processes.[4,5]

However, it has become increasingly clear that to describe the essential character of even the most casual inter-

personal encounters presents almost insurmountable difficulties of selection, summary, and conceptualization. Paul
Lazarsfeld, one of the founders of modern empirical behavioral science research, was apt to remind his students
that while there are guidelines on how to conduct a study,
once significant phenomena, concepts, and hypotheses
have been identified, there are no guidelines on how to
discover such significant phenomena and concepts; that is,
there are no methods for the discovery of crucial elements
of the processes to be studied.[6]

Interplay of Theory and Research

Lazarsfeld's reminder is of great importance in ap-
proaching the work reported here. For what needed to be
revealed were the essential phenomena and processes
characterizing a treatment program and organizational
context involving 30 to 40 professional and nonprofessional staff members engaged in everyday interaction with
each other and with the 35 to 45 patients.

All these persons are brought together within a special organizational context to effect—in the course of
months or years—lasting changes in symptomatology,
behavior, and level of disability or functioning in these
patients.

The great variety of vocabularies or languages possible for describing the complex human phenomena that
one encounters in such a setting, each grounded in a special or theoretical framework (psychoanalytic, behavioral,
biological) forces the recognition that no single description
may suffice; that no one approach will reveal the "ultimate" structure of these phenomena.

We bring to any research the full range of our experience, observations of a variety of settings, familiarity with
theoretical models in psychiatry and social science, and, we

hope, some measure of wisdom; that is, a confidence in our perceptions and conclusions.

I concur with Strauss in the view that "The root sources of all significant theorizing is the sensitive insights of the observer himself. As everyone knows, these can come in the morning or at night, suddenly or with slow dawning, while at work or at play (even when asleep); furthermore, they can be derived directly from theory (one's own or someone else's or occur without theory); and they can strike the observer while he is watching himself react as well as when he is observing others in action."[7]

Insights arise from one's own observations and experiences within the setting studied, and mental comparisons with observations that had been made in other comparable settings. Thus, even though one studies one "unit" or "case" (in our study one treatment program) the experienced observer continuously compares and evaluates what he observes with observations made in seemingly similar contexts.

The methodology involves an interplay of theory and research. It represents an approach akin to "grounded theory." In this approach, research not only confirms or rejects hypotheses brought to the study by the investigator, but the research itself generates hypotheses and strategic insights which are then systematically examined through further immersion in the situation. In this sense, the work is both deductive and inductive. Since research based on this method involves a continuous learning process, the question arises *when* one feels satisfied that one knows enough!

THE INTERVIEW DATA

Interview and questionnaire methods are frequently utilized in studies of hospitals and other treatment systems. Staff members become respondents regarding their own views, behavior, and experiences as well as informants about behavior of other staff members and the operations and purposes of the treatment system as a whole.

In my study of the High Point program interviews were conducted with all physicians, with members of the nursing staff, mental health workers, and with patients, usually in small groups. Interviews often lasted up to 1 hour, and many were recorded. Though the interviews were for the purposes of the research only, and not available to the clinician-administrator, interviewees were told that tape recording would be suspended whenever they requested it. In the course of the research such requests were made only twice, and for short periods of time.

These interviews covered a great many topics comprising the respondents' description of the program, and of their own role in it, to discussions of particular patients and criteria of success or failure. Each was asked to define the essential feature of the program and of the social context in which High Point staff and patients work and live. Staff were asked to report on "critical incidents" that would illustrate the workings of the program.

The data generated in this fashion are obviously important, yet limited. It was Mills who observed that the central problem of methodological problems in the behavioral sciences was the disparity between talk and behavior, between what persons say they do and what they actually do. Mills' comment refers to the likelihood that respondents, subjects, and informants—even when sophisticated—are unable (and sometimes unwilling) to report accurately on the interactional social processes in which they have participated. There are many reasons that explain the limitations of the interview approach. Above all, it is difficult for persons participating in a social situation to be aware of the multiple and complex processes involved. As Bales explains: "Both changes in behavioral process that occur much more quickly than the average tempo of interaction, and those that occur more slowly tend to elude conscious awareness."[8] Interview data, therefore, need to be complemented by information obtained through firsthand participant observation.

BEHAVIOR SETTINGS

Researchers determine those segments of the social context they wish to study in order to arrive at valid inferences about prevailing norms, social structure, and characteristic configurations of interaction.

For each segment, observations over a period of weeks or months is required to provide an initial description of the web of social processes involved.

In a series of important studies in the early 1960's, the psychologist Roger Barker proposed that there are natural units in the study of behavior that he called "behavior settings." These settings represent to Barker "self-generated parts of the stream of behaviour."[9]

Settings included a large range of contexts, meetings, exchanges, both formal and informal, among staff, patients, and patients and staff. Among settings observed many times were a variety of staff conferences, group therapy sessions, patient committee meetings, arts and crafts activity, organized artistic and theatrical events, informal patient and staff get-togethers, everyday luncheons and dinners, and the variety of encounters between staff and patients, and among patients themselves around the manifold tasks of daily living.

Contrary to my practice in past work, quantitative measures were not utilized in this research, except for some overall outcome measures. A variety of therapeutic settings and significant parameters had, over the years, already been identified. It was my preference to work on a conceptual and system level from the outset.

The task was to develop a conceptual model that specifies the social learning and resocialization process characteristics of social healing contexts—as illustrated by High Point Hospital's therapeutic program.

THE PARTICIPANT OBSERVER

In traditional short-term behavioral science research investigators maintain distance from the subjects under study. In past studies of hospital organization, staff and patients were unaware of the study until its completion. Caudill[10] assumed the role of the patient to study a small mental hospital, and Goffman assumed the role of the assistant to the athletic director for his studies of St. Elizabeth's Hospital.[11]

Such deception is not desirable nor feasible in long-term studies of small hospital treatment programs. Morris Schwartz, who did most of the everyday observational work in the now classic study of Chestnut Lodge, the mental hospital, was introduced to patients and staff "in his true role—a research worker interested in finding out how patients live together, how the hospital works, what might be done to make it work better. . ."[12]

The role of the investigator-observer was clearly described to staff in my study of High Point Hospital. The objective of the study was set forth to staff and patients: to learn about the everyday operation of the treatment program through observation and interviews, so that its features could be reported to the professional community.

As the research progressed it was possible to conceptualize and clarify some important program features within a more comprehensive theoretical framework, as for example, conceptions of therapeutic work that differed from those held by staff of other psychiatric treatment programs.

The Issue of Disclosure

Sharing of such preliminary insights with staff would inevitably, if only to a small extent, alter the treatment program. In a "pure" research model one would hesitate before such a step. Within an action research model, and given the small size of the program, and the closeness of the investigator to staff and to the day-to-day operations of the hospital, it would make little sense to withhold insights and findings—even if only preliminary—if they might enhance effectiveness of the program.

The importance of sharing such "findings" with staff was impressed on me by some comments of Stanton and Schwartz, who, at the conclusion of their research, regretted their reluctance to provide the Chestnut Lodge staff with more feedback from their studies.

"We had not noticed that some of the staff had wanted much more frequent delivery of information, even before it was clearly organized. These staff members later said that it would have been useful to them in the continuing process of self-examination. . . It is our belief in retrospect that the information could have been supplied without genuine violation of confidence and that in all probability such a free interchange between the project findings and the hospital as a whole would have been helpful on both sides. . ."[13]

THE CHALLENGE OF COLLABORATION

The research described in this book was carried out in close collaboration with the medical director of High Point

Hospital, Alexander Gralnick. While the work of Alexander Gralnick as the creator and administrator of a complex treatment program has been primarily clinical, my own work has been primarily that of a researcher of treatment settings and therapy processes; though I had, in the past, also worked as a clinician and teacher of clinicians in psychiatric facilities.

It was therefore inevitable that each of us held special commitments to models of illness and disability, to particular treatment strategies, and to the usefulness or defects of particular medical and social policies. It would be reasonable to assume that such commitments to particular models and points of view might complicate our collaboration.

However, it had become clear even in our first collaborative effort in the early 70s that the structure of High Point Hospital's clinical program corresponded in some crucial respects to the theoretical model of treatment context that had been of interest to me for some time, and that many features of the High Point program could be explained within the contextual framework that I had developed. At the same time, Gralnick recognized that the reconceptualization of the program in the terms proposed indeed clarified and made explicit the intent and special character of the program.

Lieberman argues that there are two promising models for collaborative research between researcher and clinician-administrator that assure the dissemination of innovative and effective programs to the professional community. In the first, "the administrator, clinician or program director *is* the researcher, or is closely involved and identified with the research and evaluation effort. The second model entails a close working alliance between the administrator or clinician and the researcher. In reality this is a difficult and challenging alliance to develop. It requires much effort and time on the part of both parties, a willingness to learn from each other, and a respect for each other's assumptions, goals and values."[14]

Alexander Gralnick and I were able to develop such a relationship in many hours of conversation and review of each element of the program. We became aware of major areas of convergence and agreement in perceptions and formulations, and also became clear regarding those issues where we differed.

Part III

TREATMENT MODALITIES

Chapter 5

FORMS OF THERAPEUTIC WORK

THE CONCEPT OF THERAPEUTIC WORK

The job of a professional ordinarily requires a special set of duties and responsibilities. Psychiatrists, nurses, social workers, mental health aides, arts and crafts workers, and other staff members are assigned very specific and distinct duties in psychiatric institutions. Nonprofessional staff, maintenance, housekeeping and kitchen staff perform different tasks within their domain.

It appears, however, that the conception of professional and nonprofessional work that has evolved at High Point Hospital over the years has taken a somewhat different direction. While every staff member, professional and nonprofessional alike, occupies a distinctive role, with special tasks and functions, all of the staff is *also* engaged in groups of activities that are not ordinarily associated with a traditional organizational role structure.

It seemed useful to describe these shared activities of High Point staff as forms of therapeutic work, since these exhibit all of the characteristics of work;[1] they involve expenditures of energy, time, and skill. Furthermore, these activities can be described and their special character communicated. While it is important to specify the "recipes" for such kinds of work it may well be that some professionals, due to particular training or personal limitations, would not be able to enlarge their role conception to encompass such forms of work.

Some features of High Point Hospital organization already direct attention of the observer to the somewhat different conception of staff function and work that prevails.

Professional staff members participate in the work of seven patient committees, some of which include nonprofessional staff as well. The committees are involved with all kinds and phases of patient activities, and with the everyday operations of the hospital. They are: House and Safety, Dining Room, Grounds and Gardening, Arts and Crafts, Entertainment, Library, and Newspaper.

But beyond participation in these structured groups, staff members contribute to the therapeutic program and the operation of the hospital by engaging in a set of activities, to be described, that I suggest represent forms of therapeutic work.

This emerging conception of therapeutic work, though practiced at High Point, is still not well conceptualized, and therefore not always as clearly understood and communicated to staff as might be desirable.

ATTENTIONAL WORK

Attentional work refers to the expectation of and demand upon staff to pay attention to the mundane, everyday occurrences of patient life in the hospital. Staff observation is not to be limited to patients' symptoms, problematic behaviors, or psychological distress. Attention is to be paid to the "nitty-gritty" of everyday existence, how patients are dressed for indoor or outdoor activities, whether, what, and how they eat, whether rooms are properly ventilated and lighted, or whether lights are inappropriately left on.

All aspects of the physical environment are likewise monitored. Concern with the "here and now" is stressed over and over again, especially when staff commitment to this form of work diminishes, as is occasionally the case. Indeed, everyone, including patients, is encouraged to be alert to all that transpires in the social and physical environment.

"No Unimportant Details"

As much time may be given at staff meetings to a discussion of what kind of prize should be awarded for a patient activity such as a kite-flying contest, as to level of medication, or the analysis of a problem a nurse was having with one of the patients. For example, in relation to the kite-flying contest, the discussion centered on whether, and what prizes should be given for the kite that flew the highest, or was kept in the air the longest by a patient, or was constructed with the most colorful design. In relation to these issues, questions arose as to how particular patients may react to particular prizes, and to a decision to honor a particular activity or type of kite construction.

A visitor at the staff conference, a well-known psychiatrist from a prestigious psychiatric inpatient facility in the Northeast remarked that in his view such elaborate concern with a trivial matter such as the contest, involving six psychiatrists, the nursing director and her assistant, members of the social work and arts and crafts staff for a period of over half an hour, might well be a waste of time. He expressed the view that such matters might easily be delegated to the appropriate staff member involved in the activity.

But this illustration is, indeed, an example of the attentional work and concern with everyday details characteristic of the High Point program context.

Jerome Robbins, one of the foremost choreographers and dance instructors, when asked to explain his secret of effective teaching—and making dancers learn—his complex ballet choreography, is alleged to have said "There are no unimportant details."

It is this orientation that emerges as an essential feature of therapeutic role conceptions and work of professional and support staff in this setting.

INFORMATIONAL WORK

Informational work requires the obtainment and transmission of information. Information can be obtained firsthand through direct observation or from other staff members. Information may concern everyday occurrences, aspects of the hospital's systems operations, or patients' trajectories: that is, patient progress, improvement, or failures. Attending work described earlier is closely connected with, and often a prerequisite for, informational work.

Informational work at High Point Hospital is enhanced by the relatively small number of patients (fewer than 42 patients) and by features of the physical environment. As already explained, the program is located primarily within one building, and patient and staff areas within the building are, in the main, not separate but contiguous, and there is some overlap in the use of the same areas by patients and staff.

Each patient is seen and talked to twice a day by a member of the medical staff who is provided information on each patient's behavior and medical and psychological status by nursing staff.

There are 8 hours per week of formal staff conferences during which information about each patient is systematically shared and reviewed. These "formal" meetings involve members of the medical, nursing, social work, and activities staff.

Moreover, it has become a pattern at High Point Hospital for the informal luncheon conversations to be in large measure concerned with exchange of information about particular patients. Staff members, professionals and nonprofessionals eat in the same lunchroom, and contributions to discussions of patients is welcomed from all present. This use of staff time for informational work is in contrast to other psychiatric settings where staff may be separated in the dining area in terms of position in the hospital's status hierarchy, and where the prevailing norm may be *not* to talk shop during such a social occasion.

Informational work is also carried out in the corridors and public spaces of the hospital where staff "bump into one another" many times during the day.

Gralnick argues that informational work is indeed an essential element of High Point staff functioning.

"Our team concept demands that everyone be as fully informed as possible about a patient's course, and also transmit this information to the team informally and in conferences. If one is to really be a member of the team, and truly contribute to its work, one must be aware of the day-to-day life of the patient in the hospital. Over and above the one-to-one therapeutic relationship, the professional team is involved in making rounds twice daily, 8 hours a week of interdisciplinary staff conferences, night duty, participation in patient committees, observing patients' behavior, group therapy, taking histories, physical examinations, working with families both face to face and by telephone. Staff together with the medical director participate in policy decisions and in many aspects of administration . . .

"All professions ultimately must learn the significance of transmitting what is important to know about a patient to the staff conference. Nothing is to be witheld and there is no private pact of confidentiality with a patient. The patients also know and finally accept this as the way of doing things and the value of High Point Hospital. In this manner the patient also becomes, in a way, a working member of the larger team. To the extent that he becomes such a member, he becomes well. If he cannot, or we cannot, help him to, he stays on the periphery and improves little. The more contact a staff member has with a patient, the more he can transmit observations to others on the staff."

It is clear from these comments that patients too are co-opted into information work. Patients are expected to share information available to them. Just as the sharing of information by staff takes precedence over the widely accepted value of confidentiality, so too are patients expected to provide information even when such actions may be viewed as disloyalty by other patients.

ACHIEVING MEMBERSHIP

A professional at High Point Hospital is expected to sacrifice some part of "his self-image, the aura of his own discipline, and the way he operates within it." Treatment strategies and decisions by each team member (physicians, nurses, et al.) are reviewed and modified by all members of the team. It is very difficult for some staff members to renounce the professional autonomy they had exercised in previous treatment settings. It becomes possible to do so to the extent that the new staff member begins to identify with the treatment team, the organization, and its values. Initially it is especially difficult for professionals to function primarily as a member of a team rather than in their customary independent role, and some are not fully able to do so.

To make the effort to achieve such membership (and to make the effort to assist others in achieving such membership) is viewed as part of the "work" of High Point staff. Rules and expectations are clarified in most organizational settings. Yet there are only very few organizations (for example, religious organizations) where the achievement of membership in itself is an organizational goal. Interestingly, change in behavior, whether of therapist or patient, depends largely—as Harley Shands points out—on the success of this process.

"The 'new' member of the professional team is accepted and slowly absorbed into 'membership' as he absorbs and accepts the ways, techniques of treatment and values of the team. In turn the team must allow itself to be influenced and taught by the new member. This must be demonstrated by the team sufficiently so that the new member accepts it as true in fact. In turn this will promote belief in new staff members that they are respected and accepted. This fosters a feeling of 'membership.' In this process, more or less, full acceptance and trust are achieved, and finally a full sharing of responsibility. A member of the medical or nursing team who retains major reservations about the hospital's treatment approach, goals or values can never be fully absorbed into membership. Such a member always remains somewhat on the periphery. If too far on the periphery, that member will ultimately be disregarded. The degree of difference maintained by each member is important, as is the level of tolerance for such difference on the part of the rest of the team. If a new professional staff member does not measure up to the team's professional standards for a therapist his acceptance into membership will also suffer. The same would be true for the new member's value-system.

Until new members achieve "membership" in the fuller sense of the word their opinions and recommendations for therapeutic transactions will not be given due weight by the team . . . The new member seeking 'membership' must realize the first and major task is achieving the 'membership,' not impressing others with exceptional qualities. In turn, the team must realize its priority is to help the new member achieve 'membership'."[2]

Trust Work

Building trust is essential to all medical and healing work. It is even more important for persons who, time and time again, may have had unfortunate, uncaring and deceitful encounters with others, including experiences with uncaring medical personnel. Getting someone's trust can be a very complex task. The task is much more difficult when the therapeutic program requires some deprivation and frustration of patients' preferences that may be viewed by patients as arbitrary or punitive.

In the course of medical work staff unavoidably inflict pain on patients, but there are—as Anselm Strauss[3] has documented—implicit contracts assuring the patients that whatever needs to be done will be done as "fast and painlessly as possible." The patient must assume that medical staff are on their side, that they will not deceive them, and that they care for their well-being. Anselm Strauss concludes from his observations of the treatment of physically ill patients in a number of hospitals that "whether explicit or not it (trust building) is such a necessary ingredient that when this vital task is neglected or bungled then patients will complain or quite literally sign themselves out of the hospital."

The work necessary to develop the trust of psychologically fragile and impaired persons in other human beings, especially in members of their treatment staff, is difficult. The patient's wariness in dealing with human beings, the mistrust of self and others can be easily reinforced, and, should a slowly emerging trust be violated, patients may withdraw even further from social interaction.

The difficulties of this work, and the problems of describing how it is accomplished—when it succeeds—are formidable.

Good Faith

Trust Work is related to the Program's emphasis on honesty, consistency, and readiness to fulfill commitments made. Any inconsistencies or discrepancies in treatment policy or in promises made to patients are, when discovered investigated fully, and their clarification made known to the patient involved.

A recent incident, from our study of High Point Hospital, serves as an example: The entertainment committee had arranged with kitchen staff to prepare a pizza as a late-night snack on New Year's Eve. Yet on New Year's Eve, kitchen staff, busy with preparing hors d'oeuvres, inquired of nurses on duty whether the pizza was really essential. The member of the nursing staff contacted, not familiar with hospital policy, agreed to waive the preparation of the pizza. Patients were disappointed and upset that a commitment made, had been broken. When patients complained (and it is an indication of the level of trust in the hospital that patients pursued the matter) the sequence of events was investigated in detail until all facts were known. Hospital policy in communicating committee decisions and honoring commitments made was discussed with all involved in the incident. A substitute pizza was provided at a subsequent occasion designated by the patients.

The incident, though minor, illustrates the importance that the program attaches to developing and maintaining patient trust. In the selection of staff High Point attempts, wherever possible, to recruit persons who realize the importance of trust work, and who in their conduct with patients (and staff) are indeed trustworthy.

COMPETENCE WORK

The ability to relate to, to interact with, and to work with a variety of other persons is important to all persons, and especially to those psychologically impaired. The enhancement of patients' social, interactional, and instrumental competence is viewed as an essential component of High Point's treatment program. This goal is without question shared in many therapeutic communities and psychiatric treatment settings. However, the strategies to achieve this goal are somewhat different and perhaps unique at High Point.

A Modality in Itself

In most treatment settings the assumption prevails that when treatment modalities deployed with the patient (psychotherapy, etc.) are effective, the patient's social and work competence is restored or increased. However, at High Point, competence work is conceived of as a modality in itself and represents a form of therapeutic work that complements all the other treatment modalities utilized.

All aspects of the program are continuously reviewed and designed for their competence-building qualities. Staff is expected to utilize all interaction activities and occasions for such competence work. Staff is engaged in "educating and training patients on how to act in everyday situations."

When patients become members of committees they

are given increasing responsibilities for specific tasks and "given a chance to learn how to deal with pressures of all sorts." Staff participation in the seven patient committees also includes the giving of direction and instructions on how to tackle specific tasks.

Arts and Crafts, recreational, and entertainment activities are considered important only insofar as they expand the potential for healthy social interaction among patients and provide for the learning of skills that are generalizable to other collaborative work situations (planning, organizing, cooperating, assigning tasks, following through, accepting responsibilities and keeping within the time frame allocated for specific kinds of work). Competence work, it should be noted, provides the conditions favorable to deuterolearning—the learning of how competence skills are learned (see section on deuterolearning).

The tasks involved increase in level of complexity over a period of months, for given patients; so that this past year patients progressed from work on their own individual sculptures for a sculpture show, to being part of a complex talent show requiring collaboration among 25 patients in such tasks as costume and scenery design, preparation and execution of dramatic and comedy skits, and the performance of musical, and song-and-dance routines.

Not all staff members are equally suited and prepared for such competence work. For example, it is ordinarily not part of the training of young psychiatrists or indeed of other mental health professionals to become skilled in instructing patients on how to publish a monthly journal. While this task may not be so formidable, the ability to communicate its requirements—in its social and instrumental aspects—still needs to be developed by staff. Competence work represents a form of serious therapeutic work at High Point.

Chapter 6

PATIENT'S PROGRESS

TREATMENT ROUTINES

The specific treatment procedures at High Point can be distinguished from the larger, encompassing effects of the context created by the total process. Just as communication both contains specific content and is the container of human interaction, the hospital engages in specific forms of therapy while it surrounds the patient with its own particular atmosphere. Here we shall briefly describe the dominant therapeutic activities (psychotherapy, group therapy, drug treatment) and, more comprehensively, the situational adjustments and role learnings that occur as patients move through the stages of development that mark their progress through the four graduated groups that comprise the hospital's structure.

Every patient meets with his personal therapist three times per week in "individual psychotherapy." This is therapy of the modified psychoanalytic type, emphasizing support and reviewing experience in the hospital context. Psychotherapy is conducted only by the full-time house staff, consisting of psychiatrists. The medical director is full-time and does not work directly with patients, but is the chief medical and administrative officer. Psychiatrists participate with the patients in the activities of the hospital, such as the committees which bear social responsibility and form part of the daily formal structure of activities, and so are able to observe the patient in several contexts in addition to that of the doctor-patient relationship. In addition, therapists accumulate a great deal of information about their patients from other members of the hospital non-medical staff through formal and informal channels.

All patients participate in group therapy sessions with one of the five treating physicians. The primary focus of group therapy is on the everyday occurrences of hospital life, rather than the patient's past experiences before entering the hospital.

The opportunity for psychiatrists to observe the contextual variability of their patients' behavior is an advantage that is somewhat unique to High Point. Rather than being subject to the error of generalizing behavior during the office hour to the larger setting as a result of being limited to only that source of data, psychotherapists at High Point are provided with opportunities to check out their generalizations through actual observations in a day-to-day setting. In this way, therapists can watch for the effects of their efforts and note growth or regression of each patient.

Most patients also receive one or more neuroleptic drugs as well as anticholinergic drugs when indicated. There is considerable effort expended to maximize the benefit-risk balance in the use of neuroleptics, and staff is alert to the development of side effects, and ready to change type and dosage of neuroleptics used. It is hospital policy to prescribe neuroleptics for severe management problems. Such use of neuroleptics is justified by staff for the patient's protection, but also recognized as a means to ease staff's burden with difficult and troublesome patients. Some of such "unspecific" use of neuroleptics, probably characteristic of most psychiatric institutions, raises ethical issues.

At the same time that patients are engaged in intensive work with their psychiatrists, they are also being guided through a series of increasingly complex social activities in the hospital. The question arises whether these activities primarily represent an amenable context in which the therapy can most effectively occur, or whether the context—its structure and process—indeed comprises the principal form of therapy itself.

PLACEMENT OF PATIENTS

Patients are divided into four groups (Group 1, Group 1 Follow 2, Group 2, and Group 3). The theoretical rationale for this organization of patients' hospital life, one of the innovations of the High Point program, is that these groups represent satellite systems into which patients are placed. Each group requires certain behavioral capabilities and emotional sensitivities of the patient, and places on him or her its own responsibilities. The professional team places the patient in the groups, each of which becomes more pressure-laden as the patient ascends the ladder to the last group. Each group gives the patient increasing responsibilities to the larger social system. In the process of going up the scale of participation and responsibility, the patient's ways of relating are tested, evaluated, changed, and replaced with more functional ways of relating.

New patients entering the hospital begin their stay in Group 1, which involves spending a shorter or longer period of confinement (infrequently beyond 3 weeks) on the closed floor. Some patients experience this stay as a severe deprivation, as "punishment," or an encroachment of their freedom. Other patients welcome this temporary

withdrawal from responsibility, and the sense of protection the setting affords.

Description of Patient Groups

What follows is a composite description of the rationale for the placement of patients into one of four groups,
as provided by the professional staff, and the conditions
for patient's progress from group to group.

This composite description is based on direct quotes
from interviews with professional staff. Since the conception of the placement process provided by different staff
members is very similar, I have combined these quotes
without attributing them to the particular staff members
interviewed. But it needs to be kept in mind that the description of the rationale and process is from the perspective, and in the language of the professional staff.

"Group 1 is intended primarily for those patients who
lose control very easily, and who require a great deal of
nursing observation, and are not able to accept a looser
structure—the suicidal patient, the violent patient, the patient who perhaps becomes overstimulated by too much
activity, who still needs a kind of isolation. They are protected, sheltered. They are not forced to make any choices.

Group 1 patients eat their meals on the second floor.
Eating in the dining room is considered an important and
desired privilege. Especially, anorexic patients are very
closely observed when they are eating, so they eat up on
the second floor. But that does not mean that they necessarily have to remain in Group 1.

Group 1 patients do not leave the building unless they
are with a special nurse and we permit them to do so if it is
a nice day. But they are under strict supervision with a
nurse when they take a walk outside.

Group 1 patients may have visitors only after the first

weeks. Placement into Group 1 is not a punishment, but is seen as a protection. Sometimes it is seen (by patients) as a punishment; sometimes patients ask to be in Group 1 when they feel unsafe. Recently two patients asked to be put in Group 1 because they felt they were losing control.

Patients are not placed into Group 1 for any definite time period, but until we are sure they won't be taking off. The question that comes up at staff meetings is always—are we now sure that they are not going to elope? Can we permit them to go outside?

Group 1 patients do have contact with other patients; in fact, we have Group 3 patients from the Library Committee, from the Recreation Committee, from the Arts and Crafts Committee, go to the second floor and work with them, bring entertainment to them, have music nights, and so on. But it is under closer supervision, so that if an individual finds it too much they can be removed from the group and can be taken to their room or to the nurses' station.

Some patients, but not all, are eager to move from Group 1 to Group 2. Some sick patients do not have the insight to recognize that they are not ready.

After Group 1, patients progress to 'Group 1 Follow 2.' Patients do not as yet have dining room privileges, but do have the privilege of participating in arts and crafts, going out of doors, going to the recreation room, doing everything Group 2 does except the dining room. We do not expect as much of them, as far as decision making, but we already begin asking these patients to make small decisions—What arts and crafts projects do you want to work on? What would they like to do when out of doors? If patients are not able to make the decision, that shows, of course, that they are not ready to go on. So they are helped to make the decision. More responsibility is placed on them as far as keeping their rooms neat, as far as keeping their clothes neat, as far as personal hygiene is concerned. It is a very gradual process.

Patients then move into 'Group 2 and Dining Room.' Here we expect good table manners. We expect no disturbance of other patients, we expect that the patient is able to wait until he is served. They need to be able to make requests, they need to be able to make choices. These expectations are explained by the physicians, by the nursing staff, at each step, very thoroughly and repeatedly.

The patients then have the right to come downstairs from 7 to 9 p.m. They have a right to choose an evening activity; they participate in choosing which television program to watch. Again, more responsibility is added. They also have a right to participate in making the snacks for the 7 to 9 p.m. patients. They do that with the recreation therapist. They have a right to help in planning activities. We expect appropriate behavior of patients during that time, we expect consideration toward others, we expect that they are not rowdy, that they do not tease each other. It is a social setting, as if patients were going out. They invite entertainers to come in from the community and we expect good behavior on these occasions, behavior Group 1 patients would not be capable of—or of sustaining for a period of time. Patients also have the privilege of staying up until 11 o'clock on Friday and Saturday night, which means an even longer span of time that they have to function in social relationships.

And then patients move on to Group 3. This phase represents almost independent living. They live in either single or two-bed rooms. All doors are unlocked. The patients are fully responsible for keeping their room neat and clean; it is defined as their responsibility. They also have to take responsibility for being members of one or more committees. The Arts and Crafts Committee, Entertainment Committee, Library or Newspaper Committee or the House and Safety Committee which takes care that everything in the house functions smoothly. Committee work is taken very seriously and the patients are also expected to meet on their own during the week, without a

staff member present to make sure that the work proceeds. Again, they may assume more of the kind of responsibility that they would have on the outside. Also, patients are encouraged at that level to attend school, college
classes, or to look for a job in order to get ready to leave.
They are permitted passes as they get ready for discharge.
About half of all patients are currently in Group 3."

From the point that patients enter the various committees that provide the structure for patient social organization, there begins a process which leads steadily to their
eventual "graduation."

Progression through Groups

How to be promoted from group to group is made
very clear by the staff. Transition points are marked by
specific rituals. Reasons for being "busted" back to a
more elementary group are also known. At times, patients
cannot handle the increased responsibilities and social
changes that occur with placement in a higher group and
so must be moved back for a time.

All in all, this process represents a replica of "how to
assume more responsibility in the real world," even while it
is conducted within a sheltered world. What is important
here is not so much the patients learning precisely how to
get along and get ready to leave the High Point program,
but that they learn something about "how to learn" in the
first place. Thus, the series of gradated groups provides a
deuterolearning context of more general applicability to
the outside world. The problem of how to generalize therapeutic context is thus approached by emphasizing the
learning process itself, and how to assimilate new rules and
more complex experiences along the way. The patient is
left with a method of solving problems generally and a
structure for accommodating novelty.

Positions in the hierarchy of the therapeutic community are determined by universal criteria. Patients enter at "the bottom" as members of Group 1, to demonstrate their ability to learn. Standards for movement through the system are applied equally to everyone. Every patient entering the hospital is taught how he or she can progress within the levels of the program and eventually "graduate." Movement within the High Point system proceeds through a sequence of formally designed stages, with some community rituals attendant upon the passage from one stage to another. Perhaps these stage markers could be made more meaningful by making them more dramatic. Rates of interaction among the patients and between patients and staff are relatively high. The number of interactional modalities available and encouraged however could be further increased.

PATIENT RELATIONSHIPS

Significant social and cooperative relationships have formed among patients and between patients. Recently I attended a play followed by a dance. The audience was lively and lighthearted. Punch was served, the music was loud, and the dancing invited involvement. Groups of friends could be seen assembled in different corners. Conversations with and among patients were honest and personal. People were willing to share their experiences in the hospital with one another.

A major event staged by the Entertainment Committee involved almost a third of the hospital's patients in the organization, preparation, and presentation. During the planning and execution of a rather complex show, involving costumes, music, dancing, poetry reading, comedy, and dramatic skits, patients, with the assistance of staff, were engaged in an extended and significant activity entailing sensitivity, coordination, and cooperation.

At the conclusion of the event, repeated three times for different audiences (staff, parents, the community) patients seemed to experience a distinct sense of loss.

Hospital norms here regarding social relationships among patients are, however, more ambiguous than need be. While patient's self-expression and involvement with other patients is encouraged around specific activities and events, patients are generally dissuaded from close contacts with other patients, both within the hospital and after discharge. However, patient relationships with other patients are frequently resumed after leaving the hospital; and how could it be otherwise, when some of the more satisfying human connections some patients ever achieved, occurred within the hospital, around special activities, and with the enabling role of staff.

While it appears that a wide range of opportunities for contact are available (informal patient discussions, cooperative work efforts, recreation, therapy) in fact, the range within these is still somewhat too limited and often initiated by staff members.

Patients still seek frequent direction from staff in their committee meetings, even though one patient-member is the designated chairperson and another the recording secretary. The activities of some committee meetings follow a strict procedure, directed by the staff advisor to the group. If the interactional skills of the members are to be enhanced, more opportunities for exercising a wider range, particularly of self-directed behaviors will need to be provided.

Participation at High Point is typically protracted. Sufficient time is allocated so that the beneficial effect of participation in the program context can make its impact. On the average, patients spend at least 6 months in the hospital, some a good deal longer. Prolonged involvement

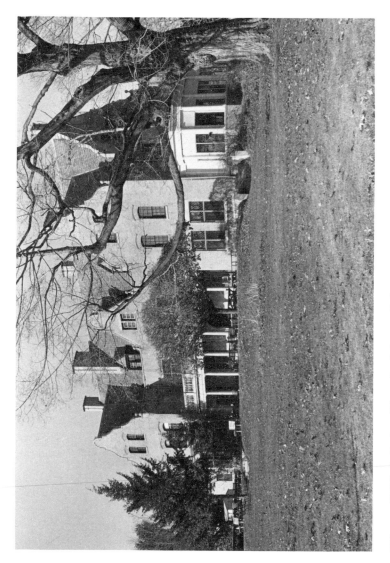

View of High Point Hospital from driveway

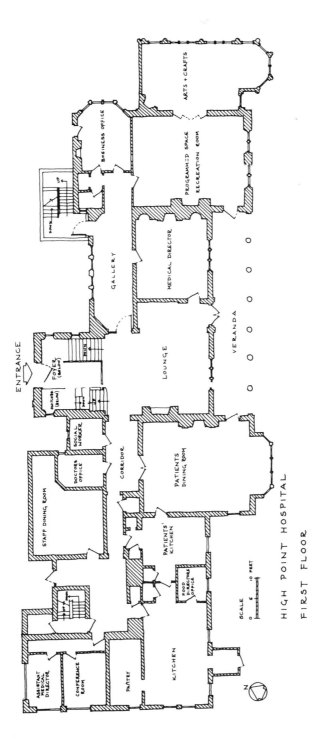

ENTRANCE

BUSINESS OFFICE

ARTS + CRAFTS

PROGRAMMED SPACE
RECREATION ROOM

GALLERY

MEDICAL DIRECTOR

UP

DOWN

FOYER
(BELOW)

POINTERS
(BELOW)

LOUNGE

VERANDA

SOCIAL
WORKER

STAFF DINING ROOM

DOCTORS
OFFICE

CORRIDOR

PATIENTS
DINING ROOM

PATIENTS'
KITCHEN

ASSISTANT
MEDICAL
DIRECTOR

CONFERENCE
ROOM

PANTRY

KITCHEN

FOOD
DIRECTORS
OFFICE

SCALE

0   5   10 FEET

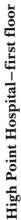

N

HIGH POINT HOSPITAL

FIRST FLOOR

High Point Hospital—first floor

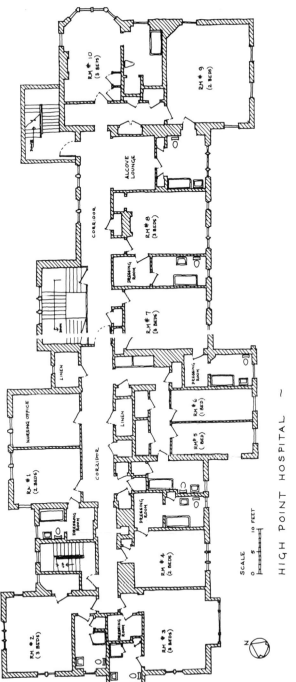

SCALE
0 5 10 FEET

HIGH POINT HOSPITAL ~

SECOND FLOOR

High Point Hospital–second floor

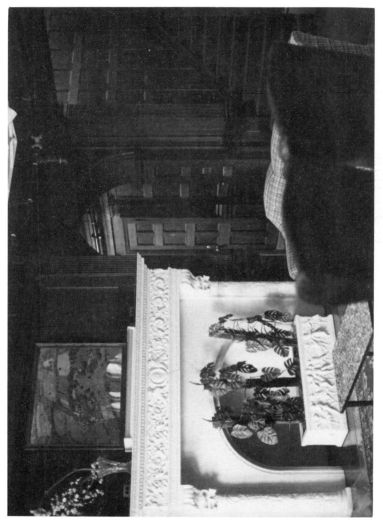

High Point Hospital—first floor lounge

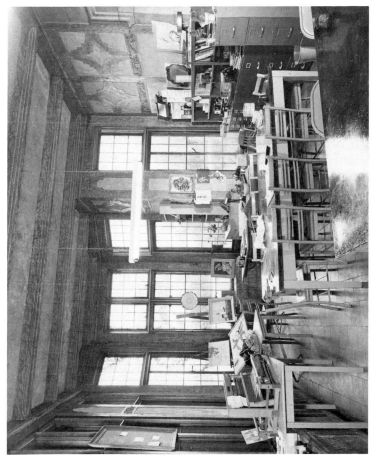

High Point Hospital–art studio

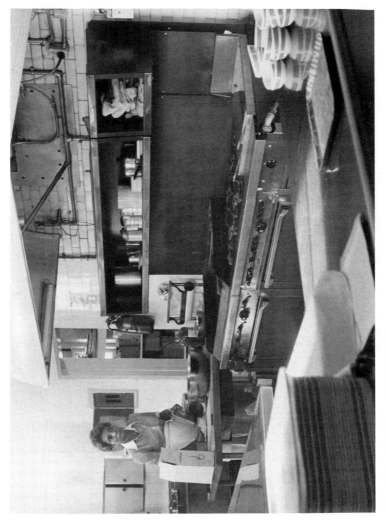

High Point Hospital–kitchen

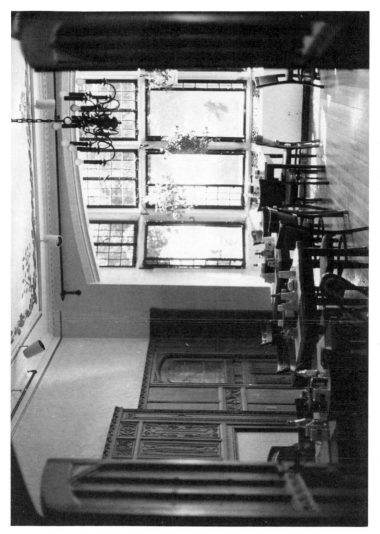

High Point Hospital–first floor patient dining room

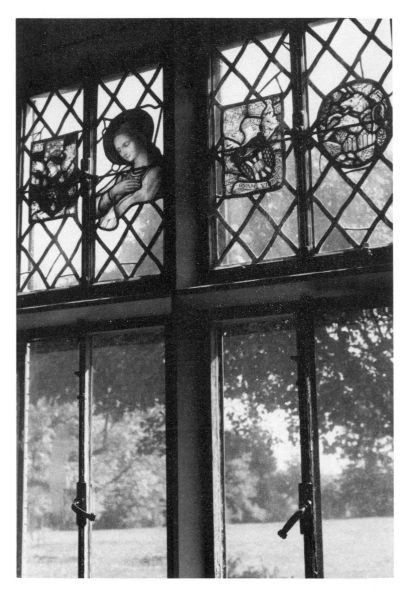

High Point Hospital—first floor recreation room, window detail

permits the formation of meaningful relationships with the medical staff and enhances the development of a strong social system among patients. Opportunities to develop new behavioral patterns are given sufficient time to "take hold." Time is provided to consolidate an altered sense of self.

PATIENTS AS RESOURCE

Yet, as already pointed out, High Point does not encourage a permanent association among its "graduates." Some do return to visit staff and do report on their progress and accomplishments, others continue in outpatient treatment with one of High Point's treating physicians. But the idea that deserves attention is to use functioning former patients as a resource to High Point's current patients, as well as for each other.

Their visits to the hospital on an informal or formal basis (for a discussion of their experience, struggles, and successes) may benefit the presently hospitalized group who can glimpse some living proof that the hospital's program may be effective. Maintaining an association may also be useful to the ex-patient who can receive a concrete reaffirmation of his relationship with the people and place that helped him during more troublesome times. Staff could also gain some measure of insight into their long-term effectiveness.

Upon leaving the hospital, the community of graduates could also serve the functions of continued support and provide a frame of reference in much the same way that the patient's family and former community once did (or may still do, for better or worse). Encouraging such associations and assisting in the development of structures which permit them is one way to generalize what has been learned in the therapeutic milieu of High Point Hospital.

Chapter 7

PHYSICAL SETTING AS THERAPEUTIC MODALITY*

INTRODUCTION

While everyone admits that the physical setting which surrounds any human activity is more than a passive wrapper, its role as an aspect of a therapeutic environment, and as a therapeutic modality is insufficiently understood.[1]

The physical setting influences behavior,[2] social interaction,[3] and self-esteem.[4] In addition to the purely functional overt aspects of a building, every building also carries a range of subtler "covert" messages. The building communicates how the user is expected to experience himself or herself, and contains cues for particular patterns of interaction with others. Generally, users may not be able to articulate these messages, but they are affected nonetheless.

The physical environment reflects the attitude of the institution toward patients. As patients gradually fit into

---

*Suzanne H. Crowhurst-Lennard, Ph.D. had primary responsibility for the preparation of this chapter.

their environment the setting within which they live is slowly internalized[5] and seen as an outward expression of themselves.

Thus, the character,[6] individuality[7] and pleasantness[8] of their personal territory[9] influences the patients' sense of their own worth and identity; a lack of barriers between patients and staff creates a sense of group identity, and the location of such barriers defines the limits of that group.[10] Spatial relationships between staff territories and patient territories, and the design of corridors[11] can influence personal and role relationships.[12]

The character and general image of the building convey a sense of the social model on which the program is based;[13] the method of construction conveys a preferred balance between individuality and conformity;[14] materials each have their own character and quality;[15] and the larger landscape of the grounds may offer facilities for enhancing certain personal skills and increasing responsibility for self and others.

Rules governing restriction of movement in the building[16] used in conjunction with territorial rewards permitting access to and use of particularly attractive spaces, reflects a balance maintained between protecting patients from doing damage to themselves and others, and trusting the patient to share some of the responsibility for self and others.

The environmental progress that patients make during their stay at a psychiatric hospital, from being initially rather restricted in freedom of movement, to gaining an increasing measure of freedom to use building and grounds, thus parallels the patient's growing sense of responsibility, self-control, and sense of self-worth.

The physical environment of a psychiatric facility thus contains many cues which, if they reinforce the attitudes and values of the staff, and the basic principles of the therapeutic program, may help to suggest to the patient ways of experiencing himself and others that will enable him to break out of his previous modes of experience and behavior.

ANALYSIS OF THE HIGH POINT HOSPITAL SETTING

Though small psychiatric hospitals share many physical and structural characteristics, there are features quite unique to High Point Hospital that are fortuitous for the achievement of its program objectives.

It matters little whether these features were explicitly planned from the outset, or evolved in the course of time. They are to a considerable extent connected with how the physical environment has serendipitously advanced program development. At High Point there is a striking compatibility of the physical setting with the program's philosophy and objectives.

It is precisely because these fortuitous features have become incorporated into the everyday operations of the hospital, and are taken for granted, that they are made explicit. When it is made manifest just how social processes are "embedded" in physical arrangements, it also becomes easier to resist possibly damaging structural rearrangements.

The environmental analysis presented here derives from a paradigm for the analysis of institutional environments developed in 1974 that has since then been applied to diverse psychiatric facilities and hospitals.[17]

Subjecting High Point's environment to a detailed analysis serves two objectives: one, to make explicit the contribution of a particular environment to its therapeutic program; and two, to utilize what has been learned in the analysis of this one psychiatric institution for realizing the value of particular environmental arrangements in providing support for the therapeutic and rehabilitative goals of psychiatric facilities generally.

While some of the features of High Point's physical environment and program (such as size) are unique and cannot be replicated in large treatment facilities, it is nonetheless feasible to offer—at the conclusion of this chapter—very specific recommendations for the restructuring of hospital facilities for the mentally ill, that are suggested by the environmental analysis of High Point Hospital.

Location

The location of High Point Hospital, in an area of family estates and international corporate headquarters, conveys to prospective patients and their families a sense of the established position of the hospital. The setting to some extent influences how the hospital staff and the program are seen: the idea is suggested that the patients who "graduate" from the program may also become equipped to function in the outside world, and to prove their value in society.

The initial visit to High Point reinforces this impression and introduces a new element: one drives up the steep driveway from the road to a mansion set on the brow of the hill, surrounded by fine old beech trees, the grounds sloping away on all sides revealing extensive views in every direction. The resident at High Point will clearly be comfortably accommodated at a secluded "high point" —a place from which it is possible to gain an overview and perspective on the surrounding terrain. In this location it would seem, the patient will be able to obtain some distance from the problematic contents of his/her daily life, and will have a chance to gain an overview and perspective on his/her own life.

Architectural Image

Many other psychiatric hospitals present architectural imagery of surgical sterility, confinement, or corporate management. By comparison, the first glimpse of High Point, as one approaches from the road, is of a generously proportioned family mansion. One of High Point's greatest strengths lies in this—appropriate—imagery of it being like an extended, but closely knit family, in which all the members—patients, professional and nonprofessional staff alike—are considered human beings who contribute to, and are dependent on the well-being of the whole group.

The style of the building is traditional domestic—suggesting traditional family values. There is a high degree of symmetry and order in its massing of architectural forms beneath a single extended roof—all of which suggest well-organized internal spaces and an orderly social structure with a highly cohesive organizing principle.

Stucco with brick detailing are predominant on the exterior—materials that are rough but warm to the touch, and that require a high degree of craftsmanship. These materials have for centuries been used in domestic architecture, and strongly reinforce the homelike imagery. Many psychiatric hospitals are built of concrete or steel and glass—modern materials with little traditional significance, and colder, less personal attributes; or they are finished externally with clinically antiseptic ceramic tiles, or with institutionally prestigious marble—both cold materials associated with other kinds of institutional buildings.

Size

The number of patients at High Point rarely exceeds 42, and there are 34 professional and support staff. In addition, there are another 26 persons who work in the kitchen, maintenance and administration.

Over a period of time patients become aware of most or all other patients and become familiar with most professional, support, and maintenance staff. Patients are quick to recognize a person they have not seen in the hospital before, and often inquire into that person's possible role or reason for being at High Point. Patients live in an environment with familiar persons, many of whom they will encounter repeatedly in the course of the day.

Public Territories

Entering the main building of High Point at the heavy glass and wrought-iron front door, the visitor has the impression of being accepted almost immediately into the very heart of the building. The glass doors allow a glimpse into the building before entering—which may help allay the uncertainty felt by a new arrival.

Immediately inside the door one is greeted by the telephone receptionist who will call the appropriate staff member, and while waiting a few seconds for them to appear one can walk up a wide staircase into the lounge. This is the central room in the building, a large and comfortable reception room, with fine wood panelling, a molded plaster ceiling, massive fireplace, and latticed windows. The room is open along its length to the entrance hall and central corridor, making it hospitably accessible. Along its southern wall large leaded windows present a view across the veranda and lawns to the distant glimpse of the Long Island Sound.

Patient use of this room represents a reward for appropriate and responsible behavior. At first, newly admitted patients are not permitted to use this room. After patients have entered the second and third phase of the program, having demonstrated that they are able to act responsibly, they are allowed to use the room on a regular basis every evening.

Adjacent to the lounge on this main floor are located most of the persons and facilities that play key roles in the program. The office of the medical director is next to the lounge. It is a handsome room, lined with bookshelves in alcoves, personalized with paintings, and photographs of friends and colleagues. The location of this office in this central position exemplifies the central role that the medical director plays in the program. He does not supervise from a distance but is close to the daily activities of patients and staff. In good weather when patients use the veranda and lawns, he is able to see patient activities and interactions, and their participation and monitoring by staff.

Territories for Patient Use

Next to the medical director's office are two large rooms that play an important role in patients' lives. The first is the patients' recreation room that is used for meetings, group activity, and therapy sessions, rehearsals for dramatic performances, etc. Leading off this room is the very light and airy art and crafts studio. Both rooms are high ceilinged, with large leaded windows, and, while some of their more vulnerable artistic detailing—such as stained glass windows—have been removed or covered to prevent damage, much of the original character of the rooms remains. The ceilings are beamed with heavy carved wooden beams, the walls finished in hand-applied plaster. The hand-finished quality of the building that is particularly evident here is a testimony to the value of the individual (rather than a mechanized industrial process) in the creation of the building.

On this main floor territories used by patients, professional and nonprofessional staff are adjacent and readily accessible to each other. Professional staff areas include the offices of the medical director, director of social work, and the staff dining room; nonprofessional staff territories include the business office and kitchen; the art studio, recreation room, patient dining room, and patient kitchen are available for patients and must be tidied by the patients before they leave. The central lounge is available for use by patients, professional and nonprofessional staff, as well as by visitors.

Unlike most institutional buildings where professional staff are given environmental privileges which convey privacy, status, and separation from the patients and nonprofessional staff, at High Point the most comfortable and elegant rooms in the building (with the exception of the medical director's office) are not appropriated for the exclusive use of the professional staff, but are available to the patients.

In the central corridor that connects these varied territories, impromptu conversations allow a great deal of informal monitoring and information exchange. Staff fill each other in concerning incidents involving the wellbeing of the patients, and the patients can approach staff casually.

The original wood-panelled dining room, with its large fireplace and stained glass panels set in leaded bay windows facing south, is now used as the patients' dining room. Not all patients are allowed to eat here. Initially, a new patient must eat upstairs until it is clear to the staff that he or she is capable of eating downstairs without causing disruption. Thursday evenings in particular are maintained as a more formal dinner when patients are asked to make a special effort to dress nicely. A Dining Room Committee, made up of patients assigned every week, serves the meals to the other patients in the dining room, and cleans up after the meal. The dining room is another example of the use of the architectural setting as an incentive and reward for responsible behavior. The dining ritual is intended as an important daily lesson for the patients: to learn that it is a pleasant experience to be served and to dine in this attractive setting, and to learn that being of service to others—by serving them—can in turn also be a very positive experience.

Nonprofessional Staff Territories

The kitchen and the kitchen staff play an important role in everyday life at High Point. The kitchen door, which is always kept open, is directly opposite the staircase used by everyone in the building. Patients and staff may pause to put their head in the door to ask the kitchen staff what is for dinner, or simply to take a deep draft of the cooking smells. The kitchen, on the southwest corner of the building is very sunny, and the impression, reinforced by a good-natured kitchen staff, is of a welcoming and nourishing focus of daily life. To obtain their meals the staff, and those patients who are on the dining room committee that week, must walk through the kitchen to collect their trays.

Since patients all rotate on Dining Room Committee all patients have the experience of taking their turn, along with doctors and nurses, to collect meal trays from the kitchen staff. This is an occasion for informal contact between patients and staff, a time when patients may see the professional staff talking among themselves, or bantering with kitchen staff.

Patients also have their own kitchen where they can prepare their food and bake cookies for themselves on the kitchen staff's evening off. Their kitchen, the original pantry between the kitchen and the dining room, is fully equipped and generally contains storage for patients' personal food.

Professional Staff Territories

By comparison with the territories available for patients, the offices of social work director and other staff offices are small, and located on the northern side of the building. While such an arrangement may be unusual, the unspoken message conveyed by this territorial arrangement states indisputably that the primary purpose of the building is for the benefit of the patients: but they need to learn certain interpersonal skills and behaviors to demonstrate their readiness to benefit. By locating staff in what were designed to be secondary support areas the building reinforces the program's philosophy that consideration of status—as expressed in office size—are secondary to considerations of the patients' welfare.

It takes a very special kind of person to accept and feel comfortable with this architecturally reinforced assumption. Persons who work at High Point must place the well-being of the patients above their own need for prestige, and enjoy the general ambience of High Point without feeling a need to appropriate the best places for themselves.

The office of director of social work is small and dark with only one small high window. However, the director of social work feels that its one major advantage—its location off the main corridor at the center of the main floor —compensates for its disadvantages. The director has played a key role in the development of High Point, and continues to be involved in monitoring the program operations.

Most staff offices are still, in most instances, as comfortable, attractive, and light as comparable staff offices in other psychiatric hospitals.

Next to the clinical director's office is the conference room where staff hold twice-weekly conferences to discuss the status and progress of each patient and to review the issues that have arisen since the last conference. It is a plain room, barely large enough to contain all staff members, but given the priority for space, it must be considered satisfactory.

Also in this part of the building is the staff dining room. This is a plainly decorated room on the north side of the building, with several formica-topped tables and functional chairs. Despite its lack of elegance, and its minimal level of comfort, this room plays an important role in fostering information exchange at High Point. A great deal of information is exchanged here informally over meals—events and issues are discussed immediately, without having to wait for the daily or weekly meeting.

An important feature of this room, however, is the glass panel in the door which allows anyone passing to look in. The room is entered directly off the main corridor space where the kitchen and staircase generate a great deal of traffic. The door to the dining room is usually left wide open, a fact that seems to work to the advantage of the program, rather than to its disadvantage. Staff are seen by patients while they are talking informally among themselves and eating meals. They are therefore seen at a time when they are not functioning in a staff-patient role, but are in a situation where they are "off stage." The staff here does not hide behind their professional role, visible to the patients only to perform their professional work. On the contrary, in the environment of High Point, staff are not preoccupied with "impression management" but are visible in enactment of a variety of collegial and sociable relationships.

There is only one toilet on this floor, which is used by both patients and staff, again a practice not found in other psychiatric hospitals.

There are two stairwells in the main building, but only one is used on a daily basis. The formal staircase at the center of the building, leading from the lounge and foyer to the second floor is not used, except in an emergency. It is a beautiful stairway, 5'6" wide, with a fine stained glass window. The main reason why these stairs are not used is that they connect the main floor to the floor where newly admitted patients are confined. The new arrivals (Group 1) are initially housed on the second floor for varying periods of time and are only allowed to leave the floor for special purposes. Group 2 patients may leave the floor in a group to participate in art therapy or other activities, and if they have demonstrated that they are suitably responsible, they may be given permission to spend evenings downstairs. Group 1 patients generally eat their meals on the second floor.

The main stairwell provides a visual link to future privileges, and a constant reminder that there is an environment available other than the one patients are presently in, and that this improved setting is attainable; for the stairwell is enclosed on the second floor in clear, unbreakable rigid plastic glazing which allows patients to look into the stairwell, and offers a good view of the stained glass window. Light from the stairwell enters the second floor corridor (which would otherwise be extremely dark) and gives it a sense of being less confined than it would otherwise seem. Since newly arrived patients are restricted to this floor for most of the day during their initial stay, it may be particularly important that the corridor is habitable, and that from it one can see one's way out to the next and better phase in one's progression through the hospital's program.

Patient Residential Territories

The secondary stairs are the ones used by everyone, both patients and staff. These were originally the service stairs, so they are considerably smaller in scale (3' wide) and functional in detailing. The narrowness ensures a degree of mutual acknowledgement that must take place when people pass each other—another example of a minor inconvenience which in fact produces some social advantage.

The second floor is a closed ward for all the most recent arrivals to the program (Group 1), and a semi-closed ward for Group 2 patients. There are 9 bedrooms containing 2 to 3 beds each, each room provided with its own private bathroom, as well as, in most cases, its own dressing room. All the rooms are pleasantly large (roughly 15' × 20'), well lit, and no two rooms are identical. Every room has either a view south to the sound, or it has windows on two walls allowing a generous (though protected) view of the outside world.

This high degree of individuality in the architecture allows each patient to feel that they can establish their own existence territorially—they have their own bed uniquely positioned in the room, a place for their own clothes, and space in the bathroom to establish their own towel rail and toothbrush holder.

Bedrooms are not elegantly decorated or furnished. Each is painted a different color, or finished in a different wallpaper, which helps to reinforce the sense of individuality of each room, but the furniture and bedding are plain and institutional. This is reinforced by the limited personalization allowed to Group 1 and 2 patients in these rooms. The environmental message conveyed by these restrictions is that the initial efforts of the patient must be toward his/her relationship with others, not to him or herself. The individual may reassert his/her own identity at a later stage, but the first lesson to be learned must be to relinquish some individuality and to accept certain general rules of conduct.

By removing physical barriers (walls) between patients a sense of group identity is encouraged; patients are expected to begin to recognize that there are others, like themselves, who deserve consideration, and that they must learn to get along with each other.

The importance of this lesson in learning to live with others is strongly reinforced in the patient's first period of confinement on the second floor, and by the rule that requires all bedroom doors be kept open, and use of the bathrooms to be supervised when it is advisable due to concern for patients' safety. At no time during this initial period can a patient lock others out of his life. While this practice is designed to protect the patient, for some patients the adjustment to this form of group living is difficult; the hospital defines the initial period as one when the patient is receiving "special" care and attention, and staff emphasizes that their watchfulness is a caring and loving concern, expressing the high value they place on the protection of each patient.

The nurses' station on the second floor also reflects patient-staff relationships at High Point. Located on the north side of the building, narrow and comparatively dark, it is considerably less attractive than most patient rooms. The comparison cannot fail to be appreciated at some level by the patients.

Centrally located, the station is almost equally accessible to all patients. It is not a glass enclosed unit from which nurses can view the corridor up and down as in many hospital ward settings; it is merely a room, like others. Nurses therefore cannot remain together in their own private territory behind a glass wall, visible yet inaccessible, while at the same time ostensibly watching over the patients. In order to do their work, nurses must join patients in the corridors, move back and forth, talk with patients, and be available.

On the second floor there is also a seclusion room. This is the only very small patient room on this floor, and it contains only one mattress. As in other psychiatric facilities, it is used occasionally for very disturbed patients.

This bare and uncomfortable room has two features that may help to mitigate its negative impact: the room faces south, as do the other patient rooms; and it is located at the center of the second floor where the patient may be less likely to feel forgotten or ignored.

Graduation from Group 1 to Group 2, and finally to Group 3 marks significant progress through the program, and is seen by patients and staff as demonstrating improvement. Each transition is emphasized by changes in territorial rights and privileges, and each of these privileges are seen by patients as attainable and desirable goals.

Transition from Group 1 to Group 2 is accompanied by the privilege of eating downstairs in the dining room, participating in arts and crafts in the studio, using the recreation room for group activities, and using the main floor (lounge, recreation room, etc.) in the evening from 7–9 p.m. (7–11 p.m. on Fridays and Saturdays).

If patients' behavior is disruptive or inappropriate in these settings, patients risk losing these territorial privileges. This fact, which is made very clear to patients, exerts a self-regulating influence on patient behavior.

Transition to Group 3 is marked by a very clear change of territorial status. The patient is now granted a much greater freedom of access to all parts of the house and grounds, and is able to leave the grounds in order to attend school, or look for a job. Perhaps even more significant is the fact that in Group 3 patients are expected to begin to take responsibility not only for their personal environment (their own room) but also for their shared environment of the hospital building and grounds through their participation in Garden Committee, Library Committee, Dining Room Committee, and so forth. Group 2 patients had been expected to maintain a minimal level of cleanliness and order in their room; but in moving to Group 3, patients also move onto the third floor, into a more private room (single or double occupancy) and are encouraged to personalize and beautify their room.

On the third floor there are 13 bedrooms, each for one or two persons. Almost every bedroom has its own bathroom. The bedrooms are smaller than those on the floor below, but they are more uniquely individual; ceilings follow the slope of the roof, and are punctuated by dormer windows.

Not every patient makes use of this opportunity to personalize their room (with pictures, posters, rugs, cushions, bedspreads, models, or plants), but for those who do, their ability to make their room more attractive, and their own pleasure in creating a more congenial setting for themselves are recognized by staff as welcome signs of progress.

In moving from the second floor to the third floor, the patient is spatially more distanced from the main floor, and may begin to experience some sense of separation and autonomy. While the main staircase to the second floor allows Group 1 and 2 patients to experience a strong visual connection with the main floor, as well as a functional connection via the back stairs, the main staircase does not continue to the third floor, and the only access is via the back stairs.

Synergistic Effects

As patients utilize the building they encounter each other and different staff members many times during the day. Often brief greetings and acknowledgements of each other's presence are exchanged. Such contacts have been described by Goffman[18] as "supportive interchanges." While patients approach staff members with a request or an item of information, staff members may also use these informal occasions to impart information to a patient.

Not only is there awareness of each person living or working at the hospital, but patients are exposed to staff members in a variety of role functions. They observe staff members carrying out their work functions, eating and socializing with other staff members. When patients put on performances for the hospital community, or exhibit work they have done in arts and crafts for a special occasion, both patients and staff become an interested audience.

In most organizations persons relate to one another within the framework of one role relationship only. It is often difficult for participants in such settings to distinguish the person from the role occupied in that setting. Indeed, classical psychoanalytic theory demands that therapists restrict their relationship with patients to the office therapy role only. Analysts often find it awkward to encounter patients in other settings. Such segregation of the person from the role is neither desirable nor possible within the High Point Hospital environment.

The informality, ease, and frequency of encounters among patients and staff emphasizes the common membership of all in the same community. Yet it is clear that there are different role positions and role obligations of each member of that community. It is also apparent that persons are in many role relationships and have an identity *beyond* a particular role function.

High Point patients have the opportunity to observe their staff relating in a variety of role relationships, and observe different aspects of their personality. One of the social deficits characteristic of mentally disabled persons is a poorly developed understanding or conception of social roles, indeed of the very conception of role relationships. Such patients "appear to suffer from a general inability to differentiate among role relationships, and to behave in accordance with the specific expectations that varied social situations require."[19]

Exposure to familiar persons in their visible enactment of differentiated and varied role relationships is an important role learning experience for some High Point patients.

Consider for the sake of contrast those psychiatric organizations where patients and staff do not have casual contact, where staff or administration is physically segregated from patients, where patients encounter patients and staff unfamiliar to them, where there is little sense of recognition or effort at supportive and affirming interchange. In such settings, staff is often uncomfortable when such unexpected contacts do occur. Such settings cannot provide the remedial social learning experiences for persons who have spent much of their lives in unstable, fragmented, and unconfirming interpersonal environments.

INTEGRATION OF PHYSICAL SETTING INTO THERAPEUTIC PROGRAM

High Point Hospital is a fairly unique setting, though a number of private psychiatric hospitals and sanitaria are also located in rural settings, and housed in well designed and architecturally pleasing old buildings. However, the conscious use of these physical settings as an element synergistic with their therapeutic program has not previously been described in the literature. What is unique about High Point is not only the character and quality of the building, but how the utilization of the building and its spaces is integrated into the hospital's therapeutic program as outlined in this chapter. Patients' access to more attractive and "desirable" territories parallels their progress in learning and adopting the value system and principles of social relations characteristic of High Point's program.

Some Implications

This use of a physical environment as a therapeutic modality is instructive for those concerned with the reconstruction and redesign of more conventional hospital structures, whether as architect, mental health administrator, or treatment staff. One of the lessons to be learned from an analysis of the High Point setting is that the quality and characteristics of the physical environment matter to patients; that patients do have preferences—prefer some places over others; and that patients, like everyone else, are—most of the time—sensitive to and appreciate a physically attractive and comfortable environment.

A second implication of the High Point analysis is that physical settings that promote change should not be too homogeneous, but differentiated in their features; that, for example, the quality of living spaces, dining facilities, and activity areas should be such that patients appreciate and look forward to their use together with others.

While it may not be possible to replicate elsewhere the high degree of differentiation in the physical environment of High Point, it is important to recognize that the experience of a differentiated environment—associated with differentiated behaviors, role relationships, and responsibilities—can be of great value to psychiatric patients, particularly when this experience of differentiation is calibrated to the patient's level of functioning.

Dimensions of Environmental Differentiation

At least four dimensions of environmental differentiation have been identified at High Point, that could be utilized in other psychiatric or rehabilitative settings. These are: (1) differentiation in the patients' territorial constraint or freedom, based on their perceived level of functioning; (2) differentiation of "behavior settings" and "role relationships" appropriate to these settings; (3) differentiation of "territoriality"—group space and personal space; and (4) differentiation in the degree of responsibility patients are expected to take for their environment.

(1) *Differentiation in the patients' territorial constraints and freedom, based on their perceived level of functioning.*

Confinement within a limited space at the beginning of the treatment program is in marked contrast to the incremental levels of freedom granted to the patients as they progress through the program. Permission to eat meals in an attractive setting, to spend the evening in a comfortable lounge, and to walk unsupervised in the grounds are perceived by patients as desirable and attainable rewards, and as a measure of their progress away from symptomatic behavior.

(2) *Differentiation of "behavior settings" and "role relationships" appropriate to these settings.*

The architecture and spatial characteristics of High Point are highly differentiated: some spaces are small, others large; some modestly furnished, others more comfortable, even elegant; some are plainly finished painted plaster, others are wood panelled, with carved beams, and leaded windows. As the patients learn to differentiate between these settings they also learn to differentiate between the behaviors expected and appropriate to these settings and the role relationships associated with the various settings.

(3) *Differentiation of "territoriality"—group space and personal space.*

Personal space and group space are clearly defined at High Point, and as patients progress through the program they discover that the differentiation between them become ever more important. Initially patients are expected to relinquish much of their sense of isolation with the attendant territorial requirement for a separate enclosed space from which others may be excluded. Patients initially must accept the right of the group, and their responsibility to the group, and must live in a setting in which the individual territory is comparatively undifferentiated.

As the patients progress, they learn that their own

personal space can become more highly differentiated from the group space, and also that group territories are differentiated one from another.

(4) *Differentiation in the degree of responsibility patients are expected to take for their environment.*

(a)　When patients enter this program they are expected to be able to take only minimal responsibility for keeping their rooms tidy and moderately clean; rooms are cleaned by maintenance staff. As patients progress through the program it is assumed that they can become more responsible for their personal space, and they are expected to keep their own room in good order.

(b)　As they progress further through the program patients are also encouraged to personalize their own room. Permission to display their own cushions, posters, models, etc. is denied when they enter the program. However, when patients move to Group 3 this new responsibility may be seen both as a challenge and a reward.

(c)　Patients' responsibility for their environment is also assumed to extend to their larger shared environment of High Point, but their level of responsibility is clearly defined in relation to their level of functioning. On entering the program they are expected merely not to be destructive of their physical surroundings (furniture, wall finishes, windows and so forth). Permission to use the more desirable spaces (such as dining room and lounge) is closely related to their proven ability not to damage these places.

As their level of functioning improves, patients are expected to become members of various committees, and in this role they begin to take an active role in the maintainance of their physical environment—cleaning up the dining room while on Dining Room Committee, ordering books for the library on Library Committee, growing seedlings and plants for the garden on the Garden Committee.

A third lesson of our study of the High Point setting and its social characteristics is that it is advantageous for patients to have opportunity for multiple social contact with staff (doctors, nurses, aids)—not only within a structured setting, or within a specific therapeutic setting (individual or group therapy)—but that they come in contact naturally in the course of the day, and are able to observe staff in activities in other than their professional roles, engaging in personal conversation, having lunch, answering a phone call or strolling in the building. It becomes clear that the environment should provide the opportunity for multiple casual contacts. In these contacts there occur brief greetings, acknowledgements and affirmation of each other's joint membership in the hospital community, and if need be, some brief information exchange, if only to indicate that an issue brought up (most likely by the patient) will be attended to at another time within another setting.

Similarly, patient access to the other members of the community—kitchen staff and maintainance workers—should be encouraged. The location and design of High Point's kitchen in proximity and with open access to both patient and staff dining areas was especially fortuitous in directing our attention to a significant environmental feature of instutional environments.

Note: The analysis presented here was completed in the Spring of 1984. Since, then, as in any program, there have been changes and modifications in the program and in physical arrangements (for instance, a gym and a music room were made available in a nearby building). Social systems, just as persons, change and grow. This fact, however, does not alter the major thrust of this analysis: to utilize, if possible, the physical environment as a therapeutic modality synchronous with the structure of the treatment program.

Chapter 8

WORK AND VALUES IN THE THERAPEUTIC CONTEXT

FORMS OF PATIENT WORK

Patients participate in the work of one or more task-oriented committees: Arts and Crafts, Entertainment, Garden, Housekeeping, Library, and Newspaper Committees. Each committee meets once a week together with one or more staff members, and once a week as a group without a staff member present. The work of the committee is achieved by patients working alone, or in small groups, and may at times absorb as much as 20 hours or more weekly. I have described patients' activities as work because aside from financial compensation, these do require training, skill, energy, and organization of time.

The Arts and Crafts Committee serves as a good example of how the committee structure of High Point Hospital operates, and how specific activities are conceived of and utilized for the purpose of prompting social competence and to facilitate deuterolearning.

The membership of Arts and Crafts Committee comprises five or more patients, a mental health worker with an arts and crafts background, and a member of the medical staff. Membership in the committee has at times included members of nursing, social work, and housekeeping staff. In addition, a member of the medical staff, one of the hospital's six psychiatrists, is an advisor to the committees, and ordinarily participates in one of the committee meetings per week. The major responsibilities of the Arts and Crafts Committee have been defined as "Learning the operation of the Arts and Crafts Department; assisting other patients to select and complete arts and crafts projects; encouragement and discussion at committee meetings; observation of and individual and group functioning, participating and arrangement of all activities and holiday functions. . ."

A set of notes is kept for each committee, recording the decisions made at each meeting. For example, the notes for one meeting read:

> Discussion centered around plans for the Monster Contest to be held on Oct. 19th at 1:30. Prizes will be given for Silliest, Funniest, Most Creative, Scariest Monsters. Committee is constructing a large Monster to be displayed during the context.
>
> Committee has been especially cohesive for the past several weeks, thanks to . . . great enthusiasm that is contagious. Second floor arts and crafts has also been going quite well, as the committee has devised simple, creative projects which seem to hold interest and insure success. Clean up cooperation is excellent and the group is in good spirits.

Each element of the High Point program reflects its therapeutic philosophy and value system, so that patients participate in a series of contexts each designed to achieve the program's objectives. Patients' work at High Point—such as in putting an activity together—is seen as having a dual function. It develops the patients' competence in achieving an instrumental goal, such as the presentation of a talent show. At the same time, the patient's experience in working with others is increased. This experience is consistently observed, reviewed, and clarified. A recent statement implies this dual conception of work: "A major, if not *the* major part of our work with patients is to help them develop their skills and to do better in their social tasks. Mental illness is really an impairment of one's ability to do the work with which one is faced in life, namely, to relate to and work with others in a healthy manner. . ."

Patient Participation in Program

In a description of the Winter 1981 Program, the staff member responsible for day-to-day direction of the Arts and Crafts program stresses the social learning function of her program. Note how activities are organized in terms of increasingly complex efforts, involving more than one committee and requiring the participation of more and more patients in cooperative work:

"We try to use all of the recreational activities as a tool for social learning, and we try to use ourselves as role models. Whatever we are doing, the activity is not that important. It's the social interaction between the patients and it's the learning of a new skill and the building of self-esteem. We try to build on the existing skills of all patients. . .

"Some of the unique things we have done: we made a "Pickle Person" competition. Each and every patient, from Group 1 to Group 3, made soft sculpture dolls. We had a fashion show using the dolls. They were made out of stockings stuffed with cotton, and they were decorated . . . We were able to get some very unique material and trimmings and everyone made some kind of unique fashion for their doll. The Entertainment Committee made a stage with lights and a runway, as if it were a Miss America Contest; we had music playing in the background, the same type as in the Miss America Pageant. We had an MC who told a little funny story about each doll, and everyone had the privilege of parading their own doll down the runway. And it was a kind of extension of the Self, it was very interesting how people chose to dress the dolls, the costumes that were chosen, male and female, how people thought of themselves. We were very aware of the process . . . I felt, at the time, that, if patients were unable to have their own fashion show, to put it onto a doll was safe and acceptable.

"We then organized a sculpture show. The sculptures were wire, wood, foam, clay, junk sculptures, anything patients would work with. We have some very artistically talented patients who felt very good about being able to display their art work. Also, we have patients who are not talented but just enjoy making something original and presenting it and showing it off; they really enjoy that. We gave prizes for that. We had acknowledgements and we had a little article written about it in the patients' newspaper.

"As a part of that sculpture show we also had the committee do a group sculpture of an entire city. The city turned out to be Port Chester. It was unplanned, but it just evolved. We had actual streetlights that worked, we had High Point Hospital, we had Dr. Gralnick, we had everybody in there, and we had the whole surrounding area. Patients felt very proud of that and this sculpture was on display separately. We invited the parents to that exhibit.

"We then developed a 'Create an Invention' contest. As you see, the activities were getting more and more complex and they involved more and more complex organization and thought. In the 'Create an Invention' contest we had everyone in the hospital participate. Patients were asked to create something unique, either practical or impractical. There were people who made an invention such as a headphone piece with two brushes—'A hairbrush for a bald man'—a very interesting and wide range of things, some things were crazy, some things were brilliant. Again we generated creativity on different levels.

"So we kept building and building patients' competence and confidence. Contests became more and more complex until we moved up to doing a talent show.

"In the talent show, there were about 20 to 25 patients involved, plus stagehands and prop keepers. We tried to involve everybody, on whatever level they were capable of participating at. It was a real challenge! We had people who were very, very talented, and we had people who were not too talented but we just felt it was important for them to get up there and to contribute whatever it was that they were able to do, and they did it! I think it was an example of how to build on ego strengths.

"The patients put on three performances, once at night for the night staff and guests, once during the day for the doctors and day staff, and the other time for parents, guests, and relatives. The director gave us permission to take it on the road to two old age homes, and an orphanage. It's important to follow through on that and the patients feel really good about it. I would say it changed the atmosphere in the hospital, because it gave patients a long-term focus, and all the rehearsing and preparing, though anxiety-provoking, was very goal-directed.

It gave the patients a chance to be seen in a different role than that of patient, and affirmed them in relating to each other and to staff in another way that didn't have anything to do with being in a hospital. They might have done this in college or school or at work."

Functions of Patient Work

The forms of patient work described serve a range of manifest and latent functions. First of all, they enhance the patients' feelings of competence and provide them with a sense of accomplishment. They have succeeded in "getting an act together" that provides entertainment and pleasure to themselves, and to their audience of staff and parents. They have accomplished this through relating to each other in a variety of roles, expanding their repertoire of social behavior. In the talent show, for example, they have worked with each other as fellow patients, fellow entertainers, yet each contributing different skills and talent (singer, dancer, actor, master of ceremonies, costume designer). They have shared anxious, and joyful moments in planning, rehearsing, and finally presenting their joint effort. The professional staff, who at High Point do not restrict their contact with patients to individual or group therapy settings, take a lively interest in all patient activities, and while being entertained, observe patient skills, strengths, and moments of vulnerability. High Point's kitchen, housekeeping, and administrative support staff, who, as discussed elsewhere, are viewed as very much part of the therapeutic system, are an enthusiastic and committed audience for the patients' activities. Their view of patients, whom they frequently first encounter in a distressed and nonfunctioning state, is enlarged.

To encounter patients in a setting that reverses the ordinary asymmetry of staff-patient intervention, increases the perception of patients as more complete human beings. In turn, these changed perceptions by staff cannot fail to be perceived by patients and become incorporated, slowly, in subtle ways, into a more positive patient self-image.

I view it important that these endeavors be seen as forms of work by both patients and staff. This is not always the case, especially for those members of the program socialized to their professional roles in settings when activities such as arts and crafts were seen as "busywork" and of little therapeutic significance.

QUALITY OF LIFE

While psychiatry abounds with theories of pathology, there has been less attention given to comprehensive descriptions of the nature of emotional health and well-being. Therapeutic efforts are primarily directed toward relief of symptoms, restoration of function, and, in a few instances, if very ambitious, toward reconstruction of the basic personality.

Yet it would clearly be useful if therapeutic efforts were always guided by a well-defined conception of what specific changes are to be brought about, and if it were made explicit just how the fabric of patients' everyday lives and personhood was to be improved by treatment. Without such a clear conception of what represents an improved quality of life for the patient, it becomes difficult to evaluate whether the goals of treatment were indeed achieved. It also makes problematic the balancing of treatment connected benefits against induced deficits. Some psychiatric treatments do benefit patients in some respects while diminishing quality of life in others. Without a conception of the broad array of treatment connected effects, and without knowing the patients' priorities, it becomes well-nigh impossible to balance benefits and risks of treatments.

That is not to say that goals of particular treatments have not been formulated, but most often in terms too broad or too restrictive to be of use. The goal of psychoanalysis for the patient has been succinctly defined by its founder: "*Lieben und Arbeiten.*" But this goal does not provide much of a guide to the kind of long-term treatment effort characteristic of the program described in this book. The High Point program is primarily oriented to severely disabled adolescents and young adults who present a long history of difficulty in personal relationships and who have been unable for most of their life to function in essential social systems (including family, school, work, social, and peer relationships), and who frequently exhibit a variety of severe "psychiatric" symptoms.

Priorities for Improvement

The quality of everyday life of most of the High Point patients, prior to hospitalization, has been deficient in important respects. Consequently, the improvement of the patients' quality of life is an objective that pervades all aspects of the treatment program. The therapeutic program proceeds from some specific assumptions regarding in what ways and how quality of the patient's everyday lives is to be improved.

These are based on clinical experience and judgments, for few are the systematic studies that have examined, in any detail, the quality of life of the severely impaired young schizophrenic patient. What human and interpersonal experiences are important and meaningful to them? What are their value priorities? What features of the social and physical environment do they appreciate, find satisfying, or seek? Clinical experience with this group of patients does provide clues about what patients consider important and essential to their well-being, though more systematic information on quality-of-life issues would surely be an important resource.

The High Point program is committed to the goal to enable each patient to find "a system of values, identifiable, persistent yet modifiable and harmonious with who one conceives himself to be."[1]

In a special study of patients who had been participating in the program for over 6 months and who were at the time of the study members of Group 3 (that is, in the final phase of the treatment program), the following quality-of-life features emerged as very important, and most highly valued.[2]

To trust others and be trusted by them;
to have the respect of fellow patients and staff;
to be relatively free from anxiety and to feel well physically;
to be of help and assistance to others;
to live up to one's promises and have others live up to theirs;
to have hope for the future;
to live in a pleasant place.

It appears that patients exposed to the structure and value system of the High Point Treatment Context for 6 months or longer, and who have made progress in terms of the program's criteria primarily place priority on interpersonal, relational values: on trustworthiness, trust, mutual consideration, and cooperation. These findings, though based on one group of patients only, suggest that the High Point Hospital program represents a hospital program context analogue to Ivan Nagy's relational family therapy contexts that teaches "family members that the key dynamic of relationships is merited trust" and the "simultaneous multilateral consideration of more than one human being."[3]

It is of course possible that patients do not really hold with these views but espouse them in the interview situation, because they have accurately identified the instructions, expectations, and values of the program. When observations of behavior confirm, though not always consistently, patients' commitment to relational values, it could likewise be argued that patients *only* behave in ways expected but that they have not really adopted these values. However, to act *as if* one had adopted specific criteria of social relationship reflects a considerable enlargement in patients' behavioral repertoire. These therefore are evidence of a considerable impact of the program context on patient ideology and behavior.

Patients do not, however, seem to identify (or think they should identify) with conventional values such to "earn a great deal of money" or "to work each day." The development of competence, and commitment to organized effort, two priorities of therapeutic work described earlier, do not emerge with the same salience in patients' value system. Also, individual pursuits and sensory pleasures including enjoyment of music, good food, having fun, are less highly valued by this group of patients, a result consistent with the well known anhedonia associated with severe psychological disorder.

But since we are all "more human otherwise" one must assume that patients also seek, at least in some measure, those very experiences, transactions, and settings that are also desired by those of us more fortunate in our biography.

In describing the work and philosophy of the hospital, Gralnick made a number of observations over the years on the "humanizing" effect of the High Point therapeutic context. He distinguishes between "normal" and "human" and is searching for a "clinical path" to what humanizes the patient. The question arose as to which program elements were indeed significant to the assumed humanization process.

The concern here converges with the quest of certain philosophers and sociologists who are attempting to identify "prototypical human gestures . . . (those) reiterated acts and experiences that appear to express essential aspects of man's being. . ."[4]

Caring

The process of caring involves knowing, and paying attention: "to care for another person I must be able to understand him and his world as if I were inside it. I must be able to see, as it were, with his eyes what his world is like to him. . ."[5] At least two of the therapeutic work characteristics of the High Point program, attentional and informational work, contribute to the caring process. It will be recalled that the basic assumption shared by staff is that "there are no unimportant details." Everything pertaining to patients matters. In caring for patients, staff "teaches" patients to care; "to help another person grow is at least to help him care for something or someone apart from himself . . . it is to help that other person to come to care for himself, and becoming responsive to his own need to care . . ."[6]

Order

For some sociologists of religion *order* constitutes a fundamental human trait. ". . . any . . . society is an order, a protective structure of meaning erected in the face of chaos . . ."[7] Deprived of order, both group and individual are threatened with the most fundamental terror of chaos (that Emil Durkheim called *anomie*—a state of being "order-less").

The orderliness and the legibility of the High Point Hospital structure is apparent in all aspects of our study. The continued insistence on the shared understanding of rules and procedures (always an uphill fight) is a significant feature of assuring such order. Order is certainly a major program focus that has been illustrated.

Hope

The German philosopher Bloch emphasizes that man's being cannot be adequately understood except in connection with his unconquerable propensity to hope for the future.

According to another modern philosopher, Ludwig Wittgenstein, human beings can be differentiated from animals in that animals cannot pretend, be sincere, or *hope*. For Wittgenstein, hope is a uniquely human behavior or experience, unlike hunger, a physiological state human beings share with animals.

Berger writes that human beings exist by extending their being into the future both in their consciousness and activities. ". . . an essential dimension of this futurity of man is hope . . . It is through hope that men find meaning in the face of extreme suffering."[8]

Hopelessness or demoralization, the term introduced into psychiatric vocabulary by Jerome Frank is a common core in physical as well as mental suffering. "In civilized as well as primitive societies a person's conviction that his predicament is hopeless may cause or hasten his disintegration and death."[9] "The schizophrenic person often says there is no hope for him" writes Otto Will.[10] There is the anticipation that goals cannot be attained, as a result of a past history of failure and defeat. The therapeutic task therefore is to restore the patient's morale. It becomes essential to restore hope not only that the patients will change, but that others, in their reactions and transactions with them, will change as well; though in some crucial ways the patient will remain unlike them in experiencing the world differently.

The philosophy of High Point Hospital is one of hopefulness; that, given time, the program can effect change and diminish symptoms and suffering. Indeed, the Hospital admits patients for whom other programs found "no hope."

Many aspects of the program contribute to this "futurity;" for example, given small changes and improvements, patients may move to a group with more privileges, and participate in a wider range of activities.

There are some clear program implications once one

agrees that the development of hope is an essential feature of the program.

For example, the model of illness or dysfunction must be such as to allow for hope (thus, not a "cure" model but one that emphasizes "living with illness or disability"); goals must be set in such a way as to be achievable; small increments of competence and function must be defined as hopeful progress; the staff must understand and share such emphasis on achieving hope, and finally, one must make sure that the personal plight and preoccupations of staff members do not preclude their communication of hope to patients.

Play, Joy, and Humor

These three features are claimed, time and time again, as uniquely human characteristics.

"Play sets up a separate universe of discourse, with its own rules which suspend . . . the rules and general assumptions of the 'serious' world." To the sociologists "play" is an important phase in the developmental process. Though animals "play," this participation in play in a variety of simple and complex forms is, as the historian Huizinga[11] has claimed, a basic experience of man. It is during play that the child realizes that there are different rules and principles governing a variety of occasions, that one can assume "others'" roles, that behavior punished in one context is acceptable in another. It is important to learn about the "'as if' or 'playful' quality of interactional encounters. Deuterolearning is encouraged when different interactional behaviors 'can be tried on for size' and interactors can, without final commitment, investigate the implications and challenge the normative rules and principles that underlie behavior."[12]

The objective of much play is the experience of joy. "Joyful play appears to suspend or bracket the reality of

our living toward death."[13] Joyful play provides liberation
and peace. In play adults regain some element of childhood.

Finally, the sense of the comic is an essentially human phenomenon. As Berger puts it more seriously "The
comic reflects the imprisonment of the human spirit in
the world." It was only recently that Norman Cousins reminded us again of the healing functions of laughter.[14]

Emphasis on these features of human existence is perhaps the most difficult to activate in a psychiatric in-hospital treatment program. The High Point staff has not made
it a priority of their work to highlight these qualities (play,
joy, sense of the comic) within the program. For one thing,
many patients have great difficulty in experiencing pleasure, or joy, or appreciating the comic. The responsibility
and seriousness of therapeutic work also militates against
the staff's focus on what might more unthinkingly be considered trivial aspects of the patients' lives. Yet I am impressed that many of the professional staff, in their informal relations, exhibit a "light touch," a playfulness not
inappropriate to persons devoting their professional lives
to working with young people.

At times also with the guidance of arts and crafts
workers themselves gifted with a sense of the playful, joyful, and the comic, patients have "moved out of themselves," and in taking on other identities in play, drama,
musical, or artistic productions, have revealed aspects of
themselves quite far removed from their usual vulnerable
and disabled personalities.

Part IV

THEORETICAL ISSUES

Chapter 9

DILEMMAS IN VALUE PRIORITIES

VALUE SYSTEMS

As we know, value and moral issues in the treatment and care of the mentally disabled have recently been the subject of considerable and heated controversy. In part this is due, as the philosopher McIntire points out, to a breakdown of moral consensus, of traditional authority within our society, and to our adherence to a variety of moral positions drawn from very different historical traditions and contexts. Some of these conflicts (as for example, in the area of abortion or termination of life) may be insoluble here—"incommensurable premise confronts incommensurable premise."[1]

Perhaps the value conflict in psychiatry surrounding measures to protect patients against themselves may be of this order. There are special value dilemmas faced by those undertaking or charged with the care of mentally disabled persons in a medical or psychiatric treatment setting. The ethical tradition that still guides our actions, certainly our legal system, stresses, in the main, the rights of the individual, and does not acknowledge the interdependence of persons in families and communities. We have not yet evolved an ethical system that acknowledges such interconnectedness and accountability. The closest effort to develop a relational ethic in the psychotherapy field is the work of Ivan Boszormenyi-Nagy who asserts that the "Key dynamic of relationships is merited trust. Acknowledging the concept of merited trust leads to a fundamentally new perspective of therapy: simultaneous multilateral consideration of more than one human being."[2]

I propose to discuss the issues surrounding values governing psychiatric treatment programs in relation to the program of High Point Hospital program, where there has been an explicit concern with value issues, and a willingness to spell out priorities, even if these differ from or are in conflict with those of other psychiatric treatment institutions.

Perhaps more explicitly than in other psychiatric hospitals and therapeutic communities I have studied, this program has, since its inception, been engaged in clarifying its own value priorities, and the value systems into which it aspires to induct its patients.

As Gralnick wrote: "A hospital community, like any other social group, eventually acquires its own value system. The conspicuous use of this system to assist the patient examine his values, which may have contributed to his illness, if not dehumanization, is another mark of the therapeutic community if it succeeds in helping the patient choose a value system."[3]

Since in its concern with value issues High Point Hospital occupies a rather unique position in psychiatric institutions, these values and their communication have received close attention in the current study of the hospital.

However, as all psychiatric treatment centers, this program too faces value dilemmas which arise from certain aspects of psychiatric treatment practice, and perhaps "incommensurate" premises.

As was earlier mentioned, therapy, as a form of human behavior, is governed by shared understandings—deeply rooted in the ethics of our culture—that should, ideally, govern human relationships and conduct. The Yale ethicist, Ramsey, puts it very clearly: "The moral requirement governing the relations of physicians to patients . . . are only a special case of the moral requirements governing any relations . . . between man and man."[4]

The program of High Point Hospital indeed reflects this position. Members of the hospital community, professionals, nonprofessionals, the patients are treated and treat each other with fairness and respect, and there is constant concern with the essential dignity of all, irrespective of professional status or state of mental health.

However, some value priorities that have evolved at High Point do differ from those accepted by some moral philosophers and medical bioethicists. Example of such differences in emphasis, presenting value dilemmas, will be examined.

Autonomy and Freedom of Choice

A major difference in emphasis between High Point and other therapeutic community programs concerns the lesser priority given in High Point philosophy and program to what have generally been considered a set of values that relate to the patient's autonomy, freedom of choice, and self-determination.

In a widely quoted statement on liberty, John Stuart Mill writes: "the sole end for which mankind are warranted, individually or collectively, in interfering with the liberty of action of any of their number is self-protection. That the only purpose for which power can be right-

fully exercised over any member of civilized community, against his will, is to prevent harm to others. His
own good, either physical or moral, is not a sufficient war-
rant . . ."[5]

It has been argued that some forms of psychological
distress and illness deprive individuals of such freedoms.
Ideally, the objective of hospitalization and treatment is to
restore such freedoms. However, this argument should
not be used as a justification to deprive an individual of
that measure of freedom that remains.

Autonomy has been defined as the moral right of the
individual to choose and follow one's own plan of life and
action. Jonsen points out, ". . . patient preferences are ethically significant because they make explicit the values of
self-determination and autonomy that are deeply rooted
in the ethics of our culture . . ."[6]

Patients' ability to act in their own behalf and to protect their freedom of personal choice is limited by their institutional status, illness, and diminished capacity.

In contrast to other open therapeutic communities
High Point Hospital in the initial phases of the patients'
stay restricts patients' preferences in the conduct of their
daily lives. Except for special activities, patients are confined to one floor of the hospital with their time trajectory
fully predetermined.

This policy makes explicit High Point's departure
from what is conceived to be a dysfunctional emphasis on
patient's freedom of choice characteristic of other therapeutic community settings. Gralnick has argued that:
"Anything that makes life easier and more comfortable is
thought of as a mark of the therapeutic community, as is
anything that gives the patient more 'freedom.' Any place
that gives the patient little cause for complaint is the therapeutic community. Any hospital that is 'like home' is the
therapeutic community. An environment that is peaceful
and that permits leisure time, pleasure, and freedom from

pressure is the therapeutic community. Particularly, anything akin to the 'humane approach' is considered therapeutic. Anything that gives the patient status and an equal
role is described as therapeutic, particularly if it permits
him to engage in conducting the affairs of the hospital . . ."[7]

High Point's norms and policies are intended as a cor-
rection of what is seen as an exaggerated emphasis on individual freedom at the expense of others, the group, and
the community. Gralnick summarizes his own value position: "My values are that people should be considerate of
others, that people should think of others sooner than
they think of themselves. This value system may be contrary to that prevailing in the general culture, that first you
come as an individual, that you must think of yourself, and
assert yourself, and be aggressive and protect yourself,
then the next guy comes. I believe the contrary! I believe
that you cannot be a humane person unless there is another human being . . . you owe that person; you must be
considerate of that other person; by that same token the
other person owes you; basically the other person comes
first . . ."[8]

The relative deprivation of patients' autonomy and
self-determination while at High Point is not conceived to
be punitive, but rather is seen as a corrective experience,
and part of a general design of emphasis on teaching an
ethic of relationship. The assumptions of such a relational
ethic are currently being formulated, as already noted, by
the psychiatrist-family therapist, Ivan Boszormenyi-Nagy,
who explains that ". . . he does not mean to propose a value
ethics . . . the science of what is right, what is wrong . . . but
one that simply states what is one of the fundamental dynamics of human relationships. It is the ethics of mutual
consideration, the balance of fairness, following from consideration for your survival and my survival at the same
time."[9]

As Gralnick does, Nagy states his assumption that the value of autonomy has limitations. For example, in a recent conference Nagy explains that the principle of autonomy cannot be a guide to relations between parent and child. For example, while the parent may respect the integrity and freedom of the child, he will and cannot honor the child's decision to jump out of the window or engage in other self-destructive acts. Obviously it (autonomy) does not work in an intergenerational context. There is an inevitable intrusion, you can call it enabling, you can call it generative . . . procreative, parenting, guiding, forming, educative."[10]

Equally compatible with Gralnick's position is the more inclusive conception of autonomy advanced by the philosopher Mayeroff: "autonomy does not mean being self-enclosed and 'free as a bird.' On the contrary I am autonomous because of my devotion to others and my dependence on them, when dependence is the kind that liberates both me and my others."[11]

The Principle of Double Effect

In medical ethics there has recently appeared a thesis, still controversial, known as the principle of "double effect." It may be that this thesis illuminates the dilemma between the divergent conceptions of autonomy discussed earlier. The principle of "double effect" contends that some therapeutic actions have several effects that are inextricably linked. One of those effects is intended by the agent (by the physician or therapist) and is ethically permissible; the other is not intended by the agent and is ethically questionable. Advocates of the double-effect thesis argue that under some conditions the ethically permissible effect can be allowed even if the ethically questionable one will inevitably follow.[12]

While this principle has not yet been applied to psychiatric treatment contexts, there is no reason why in principle the thesis should not be applicable. At High Point, patients' loss of autonomy is conceived to be in the interest of therapeutic work—to further the process of the patient's value education. In the course of this therapeutic activity, there is some violation of the traditionally held values. Application of this principle of double effect to this set of circumstances may clarify the dilemma, and provide some support in favor of a "relational ethic" in distinction to an individually focused ethic.

Functional and Dysfunctional Values and the Tolerance of Differences

Mental health personnel often become the arbiters of conceptions of normality. Conceptions of what is normal and abnormal are rooted in the value systems of the social groups of which therapists, mental health aides, nurses, and other health care workers are members, or derive from particular professional ideologies inculcated in physicians, nurses, or social workers.

There is the "danger that the psychiatrist (or mental health professional) may consider changeable man-made standards of the society in which he lives to be eternal values to which he and his patient must conform."[13]

Interventions, often potentially harmful, may be employed to make patients "appear" more normal or appear to conform to particular time and context contingent conceptions of normal and abnormal behavior.

Yet there is no cure for differences in human behavior, experience, and outlook. Throughout human history some persons acted in ways that appeared bizarre and strange to others. Often such persons were accepted though they were considered eccentric or possessed; more often, however, they were severely mistreated for that difference.

Patients who act in bizarre ways, who appear to be subject to experiences quite different from those familiar to staff, or who by differences in behavior cause inconvenience to staff and others should *not* therefore be subject to stronger and more potentially damaging treatment modalities (such as increase in drug dosage). Their behavior may be threatening to the value assumptions of staff, and therefore is redefined as "exacerbation" of illness.

These considerations are the basis for a *principle of least force*. The notion is familiar in law, as it refers to the work of police in managing social disruptions and restoring civil order. Here, too, there are no hard and fast rules of what is meant by excessive force, though reasonable persons do come to an agreement on what is meant. For example, injuring a protesting student physically for yelling or not getting out of the way may be considered an excessive exercise of police force. Police interventions are only justified by the courts if they clearly prevent harm and injury; they are not justified as retribution.

Potentially damaging interventions utilized for the purposes of management, not therapy (such as high doses of neuroleptics) may be justified only on social grounds when patients' actions threaten the physical well-being of staff, of other patients, and themselves in ways that can be clearly documented. "The recovery of many schizophrenics and schizoid personalities, for example, depends on the psychotherapists' (and mental health workers') freedom from convention and prejudice. These patients cannot and should not be asked to accept guidance toward a conventional adjustment to the customary requirements of our culture . . . the psychiatrist should feel that his goal in treating schizoid personalities is reached if these people are able to find for themselves the source of satisfaction and security in which they are interested . . ."[14]

Unpredictable, strange, and bizarre behaviors are not therefore in themselves to be used as justification for the deployment of potentially damaging chemical treatments.

Chapter 10

SOCIAL SYSTEM MECHANISMS

COMPLEMENTARITY

Both equilibrium and feedback theory are relevant to an understanding of some of the features of the High Point Hospital program. Before discussing its system characteristics, a brief exposition of basic systems concept may be useful.

When "something goes wrong" in a social system, it results in a disequilibrium or strain in the system that one or more of the participants may perceive. To reestablish equilibrium and to eliminate strain, behavioral processes must be set in motion to reduce it. Each participant in a social system is, therefore, an important factor in maintaining that system, but deficiencies in one person's contribution can be compensated by the others, and the progression of interaction can be maintained.

Hospital systems function smoothly if there is a high degree of complementarity in expectations among patients and staff. John Spiegel has provided the clearest formulation concerning the importance of complementarity:

The principle of complementarity is of the greatest significance because it is chiefly responsible for that degree of harmony and stability which occurs in interpersonal relations. Because so many of the roles in which any of us are involved are triggered off by cultural cues in a completely complementary fashion, we tend not to be aware of them. We enact them automatically and all goes well . . . However, it is part of the human condition that high levels of equilibrium figured by precise complementarity of roles are seldom maintained for long. Sooner or later disharmony enters the picture. Complementarity fails; the role systems characterizing the interpersonal relations move toward disequilibrium . . .

Fulfillment of expectations provides a sense of satisfaction and validation of experience. This conception does not imply that inappropriate demands of patients need to be met but rather that patients as well as staff learn what may or may not be expected of each other, and that an organization functions well when expectations of all members exhibit some measure of complementarity (and similarity).

Failures in required behavioral contributions, high levels of dissatisfaction, or an increase in unmet expectations, may result in organizational strain and result in temporary disequilibrium. For any assessment of organizational functioning it is important to observe the duration of friction or lag between the development of disequilibria and the setting into motion of "feedback" corrective processes. Organizational systems achieve such "self-righting" through the ability to generate information. For effective "self-direction" an organization must receive at least two kinds of information: information about its members, and information about the operation of the system itself.

FEEDBACK

At High Point all members of the organization monitor each other, but especially monitor patients and those staff members directly charged with patients' daily care. Some members of High Point staff monitor and are alert to the operation of the system as a whole. Staff members as well as patients contribute to the operation of the organization in reporting on the state of variation of significant parameters (disruptive behaviors, unmet expectations, high level of dissatisfaction, or violations of norms). When organizational "strains" occur due to failures in communications, unforeseen changes in levels of functioning of staff or patients, or due to delay in decision making, these strains are noticed quickly. There are a number of mechanisms in place that permit the required information to be exchanged among staff, to decrease the variability in system parameters and reduce sources of system strain. In some organizations, there occurs a vicious circle where deviations in important parameters become quickly amplified (deviations-amplification) with serious consequences for the preservation of the system as a whole.

At High Point, however, staff are very alert to the fact that a psychiatric hospital program is subject to quick disruption. A staff member comments:

> . . . this system gets disrupted so fast if there is any conflict in the team . . . which filters right down to the patients very quickly, and one can see the response among patients right away, they are very sensitive to any changes in this "intangible" atmosphere of the therapeutic community . . . They are very sensitive. They almost feel it through their pores, if there is conflict or disruption. At this point you notice patients pitting one worker against the other; an in-

crease in "acting out" and in difficult behavior. The key is to be alert to these disruptions and to "maintain the structure" (read equilibrium).

The following are some of the feedback mechanisms built into the organizational functioning of High Point Hospital, that reduce failures in complementarity. First of all, as we have noted, informational work is a component of the role conception of all staff at High Point Hospital, to an extent perhaps unequaled in other psychiatric settings. The acquisition and transmission of information about patients and the operations of the hospital is assisted by the many formal and informal occasions where staff encounter patients and each other in the course of the day. Information about each patient is conveyed every afternoon during change of shift, and each patient is seen twice a day, if only briefly, by a physician. Patients are seen in individual sessions 1 to 3 times a week, and in group sessions once a week. The status of each patient is reviewed during 8 hours of weekly staff meetings with the participation of all treating physicians, the director of nursing, a social worker, and occupational therapist, including a daily early morning half-hour staff conference.

In addition to the above, unusual occurrences, difficult or problematic situations, may frequently be explored immediately on an informal basis in the small staff dining room where medical, nursing staff, mental health aides, and other staff eat daily. Operative norms are such that while decisions are made by medical staff with approval of the clinical director, information is welcome and sought from all staff members irrespective of role function or status. Staff is encouraged to contribute information bearing on patients' well-being and emerging conflicts on the wards. The number of times a day staff members see each other, both in formal conference and informally, at lunch, over coffee, and meeting in the hall, and the fact that all staff members are encouraged to contribute information makes for a rapid exchange of information and attention to incipient problems.

Also, since staff is in continuous contact with each other, they are in a good position to monitor variations in each others' performance and satisfaction. Since decision making at High Point always involves an exchange of views from groups of staff members (representing different staff roles and functions), differences in perception or policy emerge very quickly. If such differences persist they are viewed as symptomatic of failures of staff socialization to the therapeutic or value system of High Point Hospital. Considerable effort is expended in working with new staff members whose prior professional training and experience may present problems in achieving complementarity of expectations and goals.

It is expected that the orientation process of staff continue over a period of weeks and months. In addition to the cooperative work experience which sensitizes staff to the special culture and structure of expectations of High Point, professional staff will have periodic conferences with the medical and clinical directors to monitor their socialization as a member of the treatment team. Nurses and mental health aids participate in in-service training programs where the details of the program are carefully reviewed. A series of papers and monographs that present the theoretical framework on which the program rests are assigned to staff members and discussed. Some nursing and mental health aides will from time to time express their interest in more formal training in the psychiatric theory of mental illness. It is characteristic of the philosophy of High Point to resist such efforts at a more abstract discussion of clinical problems. The emphasis with staff, as with patient, is on the specifics and quality of day-to-day interaction with patient and each other. Indoctrination into particular clinical theories and systems is viewed as counterproductive to the direction of the program.

We owe the distinction between feedback and calibration to Gregory Bateson. Bateson proposed originally in relation to family interaction processes that human behavior is governed by two principles, and that at times one dominates, or is replaced by the other.

In feedback processes persons correct their actions by processing information received from the human or nonhuman environment regarding whether their actions will result in a desired outcome.

In learning to ski, or to play tennis, particular physical stances or movements are corrected when one observes that the desired effect (to serve correctly, to avoid falls) is not achieved. Social actions are conceived analogously.

CALIBRATION

At some point, however, the behavioral response becomes automatic, and no longer dependent on "feedback:" the behavior is calibrated. The experienced skier or tennis player no longer monitors and evaluates behavior in relation to the objective. The actions are performed without apparent feedback.

While calibration of social behavior may be both functional and dysfunctional, the concept itself may be useful to explain continuity in new forms of behavior even when appropriate, reciprocal expectations and positive feedback are no longer expressed within interactional sequences.

Social learning that is expressed effortlessly, in new situations, can thus be compared to a calibrated response. The concept of calibration is useful to explain why functional or healthy responses prevail when patients return to settings and systems in which such responses are not expected, reciprocated, and rewarded. Similarly, patients may enter therapeutic contexts with behavior calibrated for "pathogenic" settings, and continue dysfunctional behavior despite its apparent lack of fit in the context. Like all analysis, the distinction between "feedback and calibration" will need further examination.

Chapter 11

THE EFFECTS OF THE THERAPEUTIC CONTEXT

Deuterolearning

The effects of many so-called therapeutic communities seem to be more limited than initially assumed. It may be that generalizability of behavior from one setting to another—from one mode of experience to another—had been too uncritically taken for granted.

It therefore becomes necessary to rethink what distinguishes a genuine therapeutic context from other social arrangements or experiments in living claiming to be therapeutic. It has generally been thought that the effectiveness of specialized therapeutic settings reside in the fact that experiences gained in participation in that context are helpful to patients in their participation in other life contexts; in other words, what a patient learns in a therapeutic context can be generalized to other contexts. Therapy contexts, however, must not only facilitate learning but must also give rise to deuterolearning (learning how to learn).

Generalization in social learning implies that there is something similar between the situation one is generalizing to and the situation in which learning originally occurs. Only to the extent that contexts are similar in some respects can one generalize from one to the other. Compare, for example, an average work context with an open community or encounter group. In an open community or encounter group setting a person may—by virtue of the rules governing the encounter context—behave very differently from the way he would behave in a work situation. Persons may discover that there is very little in the experience in these contexts that is useful for participation in other social contexts such as work settings, precisely because the rules governing these contexts are so different.

The Levels of Interaction

Learning almost inevitably accompanies any human interaction experience. But learning takes place on a number of different levels, as the process of interaction unfolds.

On the simplest level, interaction merely provides concrete information. On the next higher level, it may provide a first order of generalization (that is, categories). As a result of interacting with specific other persons, one not only learns about them, but can also generalize from them to categories of others who hold similar statuses and positions. But this only occurs if an interactional environment is differentiated; only then does one learn, for example, that the general class, "person," is differentiated into subclasses of persons (men, women, parents, therapists, and so on). The highest order of abstraction that may occur during human interaction is what Bateson called deuterolearning; learning how to learn. In a genuine therapeutic context patients are not only taught the principles of conduct of how to live their lives with other patients and staff within that context, but also how to learn such principles of conduct; that is, to acquire the social skills needed to learn the requirements for functioning in a variety of "real" social systems.

There is a conceptual distinction between contexts which have been specifically designed for generalizability and those that are only designed to encourage new or different kinds of experiences. The latter are experiments in new social arrangements; efforts rather to create new social contexts discontinuous from the old, and not, as one might suppose, primarily "therapeutic" in their implications.

Many experiments in therapeutic communities fall into this category. Advocates of the encounter experience and of sensitivity training place individuals in these special contexts for the purpose of getting them to express feelings and to act out in various ways. Persons experiencing these new forms of interaction were expected to be transformed by them and to assume those new patterns of behavior they learned upon reentering the old contexts in which they previously functioned.

These special contexts, however, should be viewed as ends in themselves, rather than bridges to work, the family, and to the other everyday social contexts and systems. Thus one needs to distinguish between "therapeutic" contexts and other kinds of contexts in which deuterolearning may perhaps occur, but which are not specifically designed to emphasize that aspect of the experience. Some contexts are better for deuterolearning than others. Some therapeutic communities do not facilitate deuterolearning. What is needed is a situation that is not just a pure assimilation experience.

A System of Principles

If the High Point therapeutic context enables patients to learn how to learn, then just what is it that patients become able to learn? Patients learn within the High Point context that social life operates within a system of rules and norms, and that in order to function in different systems they need to be alert to just what these principles are, and how they are enforced. Furthermore, one learns that these rules and norms concern different parameters of social process; that there are normative understandings about responsibility, obligation, and mutual consideration, or that there then are phases in the development of personal relationships. Patients also learn that problems can be explicit, and that there are verbal strategies available to clarify differences; that the other person's attitudes and behavior is often contingent on one's own attitudes and behavior towards them. Patients learn that one can indeed learn to improve others' behaviors and reactions through specific changes and strategies of one's own behavior. The continuous scrutiny and review of the microorder of the everyday interaction process at High Point by persons skilled in identifying functional and dysfunctional forms of interaction enhances the process of deuterolearning.

To put it simply: Patients learn that there are principles governing behavior, social relationships, and acceptance in social systems; and that to be able to function in ordinary everyday social situations, together with others, one needs to become skilled in identifying these.

A Theory of Dosage of Social System Intervention

Most physical treatment modalities are based on theories of dosage. Such theories include assumptions regarding the appropriate range of dosage of the treatment (drug, radiation) to be administered, the frequency and duration of administration, and the nature of the biological mechanisms involved.

Optimal dosage and duration of administration are

perhaps most clearly defined in the use of certain classes of antibacterial drugs. In the case of drugs used in psychiatric treatment there is still less consensus on the appropriate dosage range and the optimal duration of their administration for different groups, and there are differing views on how these drugs are metabolized in the organism (their pharmacokinetics).

However, there does not exist, in an explicit form, any comparable, or consensually validated theory of dosage for such social system interventions as psychotherapy, or the effects of therapeutic contexts.

Classical analytic thinking about dosage appears to have shifted over the years. In Freud's time, we are told, analysis rarely exceeded the better part of a year, while today analysis of many years' duration is becoming the rule rather than the exception.

These changes in length of treatment reflect changed assumptions regarding the total duration of the therapist's presence that is required to bring about desired personality and biographical changes in the patient. If we conceive of the duration of analytic treatment as analogous to the total duration during which drug or other biological treatment is applied, then to extend the analogy, each treatment session may be comparable to a single unit dose.

The only drastic change in a theory of dosage in the psychoanalysis and psychotherapy is that introduced by the French analyst Jacques Lacan.[1] Lacan, in introducing the "short session" (some analytic sessions being abruptly terminated by the analyst after a few minutes) did, without explicitly characterizing it as such, suggest an alternate theory of dosage of the analyst's presence. A short session of a few minutes' duration is seen by Lacan as having the potential for a more dramatic therapeutic impact than a steady adherence to the same unit dosage of the therapist's presence over the course of the analysis.

The issue arises, what "dosage" and duration of application will optimize the effects of therapeutic contexts such as High Point Hospital. The kinds of changes that are the subject of our study are of a more complex order than those ordinarily encompassed by conceptions of behavior modification. I am concerned with the "dosage" of interventions that result in enduring changes in behavior and social relationships. What dosage of social therapy achieves a major increment in patients' understanding of the normative principles that regulate their functioning in every life situation, and in their ability to apply such principles in different settings, and in changes in value priorities? We are furthermore concerned with the "aggregate effects" of a complex therapeutic context on individual patients.

Duration and Improvement

The High Point Hospital program has been accumulating information over the past 3 decades that may help define the parameters of a theory of "dosage" for the effects of therapeutic social systems. It has been the experience at High Point that the program's favorable effects can best be observed and documented in patients who have been participating in the program for approximately 6 months or longer.

In a review of assessments by professional staff of all 101 patients who were discharged from the hospital in 1984 (see Table 11-1) patients who had stayed *over 160 days* were *three times* as likely to be assessed as improved as patients who stayed for less time. Patients who stayed for a shorter period of time were about equally likely to be assessed as improved or unchanged. What do these data mean? They seem to imply that while for some patients the program's effect appears to "take" after briefer exposures (they are better "deuterolearners"), continued participation and exposure to the program for about 6 months

**Table 11-1.   Treatment Participation and Assessment
of Improvement (1984)**

		Treatment Stay	
		Less than 160 days	Over 160 days
Consensus Assessment by Professional Treatment Staff	Much improved or improved	31	27
	Unchanged or some improvement	35	8

achieves desired therapeutic effects in over 75 percent of patients. What is it then, about the duration of participation in the High Point social system that brings about change in its members?

A therapeutic environment represents a highly characteristic pattern of people, events, and norms to which patients are repeatedly exposed. Persons entering the High Point program must be enabled to function within it. To do so involves them in many sequences of situational adjustments. It is the repeated experience of making small behavioral adjustments, learning to meet numerous situational expectations, and be rewarded for such achievements that leads to a more complex role learning. The condition for such role learning or resocialization is repeated experience, the exercise of new behavioral patterns, and attention by staff and patients to the vicissitudes of this process. An additional element is the timing of level of difficulty inherent in the behavioral demands made upon patients. The social living situations in which patients are placed vary in difficulty and patients differ in their ability to respond. The High Point Hospital program as a whole, as well as each distinct part of the program, is organized in terms of levels of difficulty.

Synergistic Effects

Yet it would be an error to view the level of social learning that occurs as simply incremental. Rather, we hold with Shands' imaginative suggestion that social instructions, the social equivalent of treatment dosage, may be analogous in their effect to that of viruses.[2] Just as viruses may lie dormant within the organism, to become active only under certain specified circumstances, so likewise will information about appropriate role behaviors, received or experienced in interaction with therapist, nursing staff, or other patients, lie dormant and not be acted on until other conditions have been met. Those may include repeated experience in a variety of settings, repeated clarifications of the demands involved, absence of noxious or destructive communications, and the development of trust in the program and its staff. Furthermore, interactional experiences and role instructions in a variety of settings (living, social, instrumental) may exert a synergistic effect[3] so that there is a jump or increment in behavioral change that goes beyond the simple additive impact of individual experiences.

This process may be quite familiar to those engaged in the teaching of languages or of the physically handicapped where similar synergistic learning seems to occur.

Conceptions of "how long" treatment needs to last to effect specific changes varies with the condition or problem. In the rehabilitation of polio patients, patients and parents thought of progress in terms of weeks, and were disturbed if they could not observe measurable progress in restoration within a short time. Staff, on the other hand, were pleased with minor improvements in patient's physical state that occurred within months.[4]

A still more dramatic example is provided by the now classic work of Julius Roth on the timetable of the tuberculosis patient. Roth describes the disparity in expectations between TB sanitarium staff and the incoming patients (and their families) about how soon significant progress in the arrest or cure of the disease was to be expected. The differences in time perspectives were considerable. Patients, after a time, become in fact socialized to the time perspective of sanitarium staff who evaluate progress in terms of months.[5] Indeed, it is claimed that patients who are best able to adapt to the time frame of the institution may fare the best medically. The model of physical rehabilitation may, therefore, be clearly relevant to the work task of a therapeutic context.

Sometimes a patient will be slow in making progress from the point of view of some staff members and they may advocate discharge or transfer to another "less ambitious" setting. If a different "time" perspective prevails, and the patient is encouraged to stay and to continue participation in the program, then useful changes, at an accelerated pace, may be demonstrated in some patients.

The optimal duration of participation in the High Point therapeutic program no doubt varies with patient status, characteristics, and previous life experiences. But clearly the position of duration of treatment differentiates High Point from other treatment settings, indeed from current medical and social policies on psychiatric hospitalization. The High Point experience is also compatible with a view of psychological disability as, perhaps, a partly intractable condition.[6] (See Appendix, "A Conception of Mental Disorder.") But while the condition or disease may not be "curable," the massive secondary effect may be reversed through participation in a complex social context designed as a human learning environment. As do other learning and regenerative processes, social therapy requires time and repeated experience.

CRITERIA FOR PATIENT CHANGE

This book is not an outcome study in the sense the term is usually understood. Outcome studies often inventory a variety of procedures and treatments used but fail to identify just what actually transpires within a program. It becomes difficult, if not impossible, to identify which features of the treatment environment are connected with particular outcomes. As Ellsworth points out in a recent review of studies purporting to measure the "effectiveness of treatment environments," the major area in need of attention is the "linking of treatment process or program characteristics with outcome effectiveness." It means little for investigators to claim that they were measuring the effects of "milieu" treatments when they do not describe features of the physical and social context of such treatments. The term "milieu treatment" has become so generalized, notes Ellsworth, that "it means different things to different people."

This is not the case in our study. Role conceptions and behaviors are clearly delineated and interactional processes characteristic of the therapeutic context of the High Point Hospital program are clearly described.

The structures and main features of the program itself, the placement of patient into groups, the differential access to physical space, the increased participation in patient work, reflect the assumption that most patients, irrespective of symptomatology and disability, can and do change and make progress, though within different time frames. For example, 73 percent of patients who stayed in the program over 100 days in 1984 progressed through the four phases of the program and were discharged as members of Group 3. Membership in Group 3, as described earlier, reflects the ability to assume responsibility for most facets of daily life, participate in committee work, have access to all hospital territories, evenings and weekends, attend school, look for work, visit with family.

Group 3 patients also identify, or report that they identify with the relational values that characterize the hospital value structure. Membership in Group 3 in itself is prima facie evidence that more serious symptomatology such as delusions, hallucinations, and paranoid features have abated or are much diminished.

The reorganization of the social world in value terms and the diminution of symptoms reflect a more functional coping, irrespective of the perhaps continuing patient vulnerability.

Finally, the model of social therapy exemplified by the High Point program has been shown to be congruent with major recent contributions of social science theory to the understanding of processes of social learning, resocialization, and deuterolearning.

EPILOGUE

I have presented a framework for an understanding of a treatment context conducive to behavioral, attitudinal and value change. Situational adjustment, deuterolearning, resocialization and social control were among the concepts most suitable to describe the configuration of social interaction processes characteristic of such a context. Characteristic of the treatment program, too, were expanded conceptions of therapeutic role and therapeutic work, and an explicit concern with values and the quality of everyday life. It was also essential to the program's effectiveness that the design of the program's physical setting reinforce its therapeutic premises. All these elements form the basis for the theory of dosage of therapeutic intervention outlined in the book. The study of the High Point Hospital program then provided the opportunity to illustrate, in considerable detail, each of these facets of therapeutic context and process.

If it has not already become apparent, I now stress that the model I have described and illustrated in *The Psychiatric Hospital* is by no means limited to the one psychiatric inpatient facility studied in depth here, but indeed, has wider significance for the design of a range of psychiatric and rehabilitation programs that aim to influence symptoms, behavior and values through the creation of specially structured contexts.

The model outlined here is pertinent to the organization of treatment programs for such diverse populations as alcoholic persons and those with drug problems, and has bearing on a host of issues faced in rehabilitative work with persons with chronic physical disabilities.

For all of the populations enumerated above—as for the patients in the High Point Hospital program—the social, learning, attitudinal and value consequences arising from the antecedent deficit or disability (diseases, if you will) represent the major obstacle to patients' enhanced personal functioning and social integration. Some of the consequences range from failures of social learning, dysfunctional values, to erroneous epistemologies of social behavior (see Appendix 3).

The variety of elements and processes described in *The Psychiatric Hospital* are seen as essential for any treatment program attempting to achieve change and to provide persons with social skills, competencies and value orientations indispensable to social survival and to living with a measure of dignity and satisfaction, given the limits imposed by illness or disability.

Indeed, some of the psychiatric and rehabilitative treatment contexts that I have observed over the years already exhibit a number of the features here described. In this work, however, I have endeavored to make explicit–to those concerned with contexts that effect change–the theoretical foundation of their work, and provided a mosaic of the interconnected and essential elements to be incorporated into the design of any effective treatment context.

Though the analysis presented in this book is often

concrete and particular, it will, I believe, contribute in tangible ways to the difficult, but much needed, integration of clinical and behavioral science perspectives on the relation between social context, behavioral process, and therapeutic change.

Part V

APPENDICES

A CONCEPTION OF MENTAL DISORDER

It is a sobering experience to reread Emil Kraepelin's *One Hundred Years of Psychiatry* and learn of psychiatric treatments popular in the 19th century, such as the use of nausea and hollow wheel treatments, of masks, bulbs, and the revolving chair.[1] But more disturbing perhaps are the conviction and certainty with which these treatments were applied and justified. "Those who forget history are destined to relive it" is a statement attributed to Nietzsche. It is valuable to remind ourselves of the foibles and errors of the past, distasteful as it may be, if only to reduce the human propensity for certainty. Bateson, a close observer of the healing profession for most of his life, wrote, "Suffering is the inevitable product of action combined with ignorance . . . the matter is simple! We are all deeply ignorant and there can be no competition in ignorance."[2]

The practitioner, the therapist, medical or nonmedical, is always committed to action, to applying the latest technique, drug, or gadget in response to the pressures to get something done. Thus the practitioner serves as an agent of a cultural ideology that sees all problems, human or otherwise, as subject to rapid solution, preferably by technological means.

Time and time again, we are alerted, in all spheres of life, to major "breakthroughs," and made to believe we will ultimately solve all problems. An American scientist widely known for his cancer research is reported to have said that we are on the threshold of engineering human cells so that none of the things we now call "disease" need exist at all.

A belief in "progress," Irv Zola notes, is "part and parcel of a series of value orientations . . . an orientation of man over nature, including his own nature and biology. Thus there is no river that cannot be tamed, no mountain that cannot be leveled, no force of nature that cannot be harnessed, and no disease or symptom that cannot be cured or at least treated."[3]

One aspect of such therapeutic optimism, whether in medicine generally or psychiatry, is denial—the denial that there are mysteries never to be fathomed and persons who, perhaps, cannot be "cured"—at least not in terms of what is commonly understood by that term.[4]

To resist cure, not to be "normal," that is, not to be like everyone else, led—in the not too distant past—to the many horrors committed in the name of treatment. Yet even today, it is the intractable, the person who is different in experience and behavior who is still an irresistible attraction to the pharmaceutical industry and to therapists of all persuasions. A promise of cure is always held out, and finds its "true believers." Sooner or later, though, these will transfer their enthusiasm to another miracle drug or to another "new" therapy modality. Professionals and laypeople feel the need to assure and to be reassured that something can and will be done for the mentally disabled and that we are indeed in control of the unique and the unpredictable.

Views of the phenomenon of mental disorder, or descriptions of the human condition of schizophrenia, have been widely divergent in the past and are so today. Indeed, the history of psychiatry lives in the present, not only in the past. The human troubles, disabilities, impairments, vulnerabilities, or illnesses classified and re-classified for a variety of purposes (the latest are mainly actuarial!) have been "looked upon as indications of devil possession, personal wickedness, divine punishment, revelations of great truth, malingering, genetic-constitutional defects, 'classical' disease of the nervous system, disorders of a vaguely defined mind, biochemical lacks or irregularities, and so on"[5] and as Otto Will writes "Treatment theories have been as variable as the theories of etiology . . . neither the disease nor the mystery were done away with by the treatments used or the explanations offered in their support. Removal of supposed foci of infection, the use of barbiturates in prolonged "sleep," leukotomy, ataractic drugs; I witnessed the practice or results of all these and was impressed by the fragile—if any—connection between the treatments and the possible nature of the disorder."[6]

Even moral philosophers concerned with the rights of the "mentally ill" take for granted popular assumptions advanced by some psychiatrists—that mentally ill persons, as a group, cannot be viewed as autonomous persons; that they are potentially violent (a few are); and that most are tormented by the recognition of their difference (some are, some are not).

To clarify the experience of mental illness a conception of social and medical iatrogenesis is needed. Such a conception would do justice to the observation that much distress of patients arises from the fear of being "mentally ill"; from the fear—a very real one—of what may and does happen to persons so described. As Harley Shands asserted, "Descriptions are Prescriptions."

Contact with the Mental Health System brings a patient into contact with many persons with a narrow view of what is "normal," with persons who are themselves agents of a special conception of suitable life-styles, often exhibit little tolerance for difference, and exercise considerable power over one's fate.

The settings and institutions into which patients are placed (except for some notable exceptions) often involve deprivation of liberty, narrowing of choices and possibilities of self-care, and little opportunity for useful social learning.

Current treatment with neuroleptic drugs implies a reduced quality of life for most patients and some drug-induced impairments of social competence, and physical side effects (akathesias, dystonias, etc.).

Looking for etiology in individuals and a treatment focus on an individual's "disease" also works against what is most needed to enable mentally disabled persons to live in the community and to enable others to live with them.

Irrespective of the etiology of their condition or illness, these persons require, like all of us, adequate arrangements for housing, rest, protection, support, and the opportunity to be with others, or by oneself, depending on one's preference and state of mind.

I assume that there are, and always will be, persons more vulnerable, more sensitive, confused, and prone to inferences divergent from those of "normal" persons. Among such different persons, too, the salience of issues of hope and despair, approach and isolation, esteem and lack of it, justice and lack of it, may be different than for most of us. Their value system thus may have a different structure and organization. Such a conception seems entirely consistent with genetic studies and the "discovery" of a range of differences in biochemical, information processing, and other organismic parameters.

An exclusively biological conception of mental illness, however, has—in the past— become associated with, and been used to justify potent and invasive modalities: lobotomy, insulin and electric shock treatments, and the use of powerful neuroleptic agents. It has also led to desperate experiments such as the LSD experiments of the 1950s, for which, to say the least, a moral consensus was lacking. I have already referred to the psychiatric treatments of the 19th century. These treatments, however, as odd as they sound today, did not have the potential for the far-reaching, long-range damage that contemporary technological treatments do.

The most prevalent form of treatment today, treatment with neuroleptic drugs, may result in very serious long-range side effects and disorders. The idea that such potent intervention does not have serious adverse outcomes was a hope that psychiatrists clung to for a long time, but that has finally proven false. Some patients, in their own view, and that of their families and physicians, are thought to benefit from a short-range, careful use of neuroleptic agents, and alertness to the risk-benefit equation.

But, overall, the current model of schizophrenia as a biological illness, and a preoccupation with physical treatment modalities entails serious physical consequences for many patients, about which there has been rationalization and acquiescence (for instance the estimated prevalence of Tardive Dyskinesia, a serious neurological disorder associated with the long-term use of neuroleptic agents is at least 20 to 30 percent).[7]

There are additional untoward consequences of the current conception. It offers to patients, their families, and the community the hope that the experts will provide a simple solution that will solve the problem of schizophrenia just as that of pneumonia, that indeed there will be a magic-bullet cure for this complex human condition.

This view further perpetuates the sense of strangeness and fear of persons who are different. Such persons were formerly viewed as possessed by the devil and are now seen as possessed by an illness. Many of the mentally disabled themselves share this view.

Most of the social institutions, with some exceptions, developed to contain, and care for the mentally ill, en masse, have themselves created additional secondary problems. About the settings developed for persons released from hospitals—single-room occupancy hotels, nursing homes, adult homes, and so-called "family care facilities" there is little good news. The quality of everyday life in most of these places is minimal.

I would like to propose a different conception of mental disorder: one that is implicit in the views and works of such diverse scholars as Michael Foucoult, Carl Gustav Jung, Ludwig Wittgenstein, Gregory Bateson, and Stephen Toulmin. Thoughtful students of schizophrenia, including Frieda Fromm-Reichman,[8] Sylvano Arieti,[9] Ted Lidz,[10] L. Ciompi[11] and Otto Will[12] have, over the years, expressed similar views. What then are the elements of this conception?

It is based on the realization that throughout human history there have been persons who experienced the social world quite differently from most other persons; who could be characterized as more vulnerable, sensitive, disordered, subject to transient or enduring ideas that they found terrifying or inspiring; that such persons were unable to share the meaning structure of their contemporaries, that is, unable to conform or to act predictably.

Such persons were characterized by others as bizarre, mad, possessed, troublesome, or mentally ill. Among these there have been some who were designated, and accepted the designation of witches. But also among them we find religious leaders and great artists (Van Gogh, Hoelderlin, and Schumann to name just a few). For most such persons, however, there was little to compensate for the disordered personal experience and the associated deficits in social functioning.

At most times and places the explanation of these "differences" (whether in moral or medical terms) and the "intractability" of these differences led to social policies and treatment procedures now acknowledged as tragic. There have been other characterizations of persons called schizophrenic or crazy that are likely to yield more benign consequences. Larry Gostin, legal counselor for the British Mental Health Association (Mind) speaks of a *Human Condition*.[13] Wittgenstein, in a letter to his student, Drury, who became a psychiatrist, suggests that in the schizophrenic one is faced with persons committed to a different *Lebensform*;[14] and Gregory Bateson writes that if the term schizophrenic is to be used at all, then it is to refer to a "definable aggregate of formal characteristics of personal interaction".[15] We also need to be mindful of Fromm-Reichman's admonition that: "The recovery of many schizophrenics depends on the psychotherapist's freedom from conventional attitudes and prejudices. These patients cannot and should not be asked to accept guidance toward a conventional adjustment. Schizophrenia, in this sense, is not an illness but a specific state of personality with its own ways of living . . ."[16] And while we thus acknowledge the fact of a difference, in experience and behavior, that distinguishes some of our fellow human beings, as mental health professionals we can also never forget that "everyone is much more simply human than otherwise."

There may be many reasons and sources for a different state of personality and way of living; genetic, neurophysiological, biochemical, psychological, ecological, social, familial, including family interaction patterns and double binds.

Human difference may also be validated, reinforced,

and fixed by the reactions, attitudes, and behavior of other persons, and by procedures and policies of social and medical management of such persons (fear, contempt, rejection, isolation, forced treatment). Labeling Theory, as developed by Lemert[17] and Scheff[18] describes the dynamics of the process of such secondary iatrogenesis.

In describing such different persons—schizophrenics, if you will—as chronically or mentally ill, social resources become available for their care and management. Their medical treatment becomes reimbursable and social support systems—though often woefully inadequate— are legitimized. But their description in exclusively medical terms has serious disadvantages as well. They become a problem for professionals alone. Attention is focussed on the "ill" person, treatment, and a hope for cure. And equal, if not more important, objectives are neglected.

Among issues that would receive higher priority within the alternative conception proposed here are:

> how can social contexts be structured in which schizophrenic persons gain increased social and instrumental competence, and sensitivity to rules of interpersonal conduct (deuterolearning) and social survival values;
>
> how can such persons, given their different mode of being and experience, be assured of a life of satisfactions, dignity, and enjoyment; how can the sense of rejection and isolation often felt by such persons be reduced;
>
> how may their families be assisted to live with what they perceive to be unpredictable and troublesome persons; what resources may be provided to families to lessen their emotional and economic burdens;
>
> how can the fear and contempt of persons in the community of such persons be diminished; how can the

community be assisted to "live with or next to" unpredictable, strange and different persons;

how can we expand the mental health professionals' conception of what is acceptable behavior and way of living; and to include in their conception of care a recognition of their patients' different "*Lebensform;*" and to exercise restraints in the use of chemical controls to force conformity.

I suggest that questions arising from this alternative conception of mental disorder—as a different state of personality or being not curable but, under favorable conditions compatible with a measure of social participation— deserve serious and immediate attention.

Appendix 2

PARADIGM FOR AN ANALYSIS OF THE PHYSICAL ENVIRONMENT OF A PSYCHIATRIC HOSPITAL

The analysis of the significance of the physical environment of High Point Hospital is based on a systematic method for analyzing a building's meaning to its users. This method involves systematic observation, objective description of the physical environment, and identification of the meanings and connotations of each described element in the environment.

The following paradigm summarizes all aspects of the environment that must be considered if a thorough and comprehensive analysis is to be made. The paradigm is divided into sections that deal with the physical environment as it would be experienced by the different user-groups in the hospital (patients, professional and non-professional staff, visitors) and by outsiders.

Each section in the paradigm is structured as a series of questions that must be answered by objective descriptive statements.

This is a method of analysis developed by Suzanne H. Crowhurst-Lennard, Ph.D., in 1972, at the University of California, Berkeley, Department of Architecture. The approach incorporates concepts developed by researchers in the field of man-environment studies—concepts such as "territory, boundary, and orientation," "personal space," "interactional setting," "centrifugal and centripetal space," "territorial unit," "architectural symbolism," "architectural metaphor," and "internalization." These concepts are implied in the questions asked in the paradigm.

The first application of this method of architectural analysis was in the study of the fit between family home environment and family interaction. ("A House is a Metaphor," in *Journal of Architectural Education*, 1974 Vol. XXVII, No. 2, 3, pp. 35-53; and "Architecture: Effect of Territory, Boundary and Orientation on Family Functioning," in *Family Process*, Vol. 16, No. 1 (March 1977, pp. 49-66.)

This method was subsequently applied to the analysis of institutional settings such as psychiatric hospitals, alcoholism and drug detoxification and rehabilitation centers, and community mental health centers.

1. The Hospital as a Whole from the Outside

The neighborhood. Where is the hospital located; in what social sector of town; what kind of facilities are nearby; what is the general tenor of the neighborhood; what are the "basic assumptions" of the neighborhood as evident in the environment; what does the neighborhood suggest about the general character of the hospital?

Orientation and boundary: relation of hospital to immediate neighborhood: Is the hospital on a major street, a dead-end street; can it be seen from far away; what view does one get of it; is it set back from the road; surrounded by a high wall; what do these relationships suggest about the assumed relationship between the neighborhood and the hospital?

External image: Is the building large or small, imposing or homely, new or old, in good repair or needing attention, colorful or somber; are the windows large, the entrance easily visible; are the building materials impervious or well-weathered?

What do all these qualities suggest about the character of the hospital as whole?

2) THE HOSPITAL AS EXPERIENCED BY THE PATIENT

2a) Crossing the Threshold

Is the entrance visible or hidden from view; is it wide and well lit, or small and dark; is there a porch or canopy to provide shelter from wind and rain; does the entrance lead directly into the central, most important or key areas in the hospital, or does it lead into a part of the hosptial of minor or secondary significance? Is this entrance welcoming or forbidding, straightforward or obscure? What initial impression concerning the hospital's attitude towards the patient is the patient likely to receive while entering the hospital?

In what setting is the patient formally inducted into the hospital: for example, is it a bare, white, antiseptic hospital-like setting; a formal businesslike office; or a more informal, personalized, book-lined study? What messages are conveyed by the setting about the fundamental character of the program, and the patient-staff relationships?

2b) Personal Patient Territories

Note: If the patient is expected to occupy two or more consecutive "personal territories" during different phases of his/her stay at the hospital, the following analysis should be undertaken for each phase setting. Such a comparative analysis is most important, because the patient is likely to interpret his/her progress through the program to some extent as a function of the messages conveyed by these different physical settings.

Territory: What constitutes the patient's personal territory—bed, closet, drawers, shelves, pinboard, etc.? Is it comfortable or bare; does it have any unique attributes that make it easily identifiable, or is it identical to all other patient territories? What colors, textures, furnishings, and lighting comprise this personal territory, and what do these elements say about the assumed character or identity of the patient? To what degree can the patient make this his/her territory, personalize the space; to what extent and after what period of time; and what does this say about the assumed degree of personal investment the patient should put into the hospital? What messages are conveyed by the setting assigned as the patient's personal territory?

Boundary: What boundary conditions exist around the patient's personal territory, and how does this territory relate to other spaces? Is the patient's bed in a dormitory or ward, a private room, or a room shared with others; are there partitions or walls separating patients, or between patients and staff, and do these create spatial, visual, or aural boundaries?

What do these boundary conditions suggest about the patient's relationship to other patients or staff? And what do they suggest is the chosen balance between patient's privacy and necessity for supervision?

Orientation: Is the furniture (bed, chair) within the private territory arranged so that the patient faces toward other patients or staff in the room, or is it oriented away from others, toward a wall or window: how is the room connected to staff territories and to the rest of the building, and how is this connection modified by size and design of door, length of corridor, locked doors, etc.? How is the room oriented in relation to the outside world (the view, sun) and how is this relationship modified by size and design of windows, existence of bars, and so forth? What do these orientation characteristics suggest is the appropriate attitude of the patient to the program and to the outside world?

2c) "Therapeutic Territories:" Spaces Experienced by the Patients and Staff Engaged in "Therapeutic Interaction"

Note: In some psychiatric hospitals, "therapeutic interaction" may be considered to take place within limited structured situations only—that is, in individual or group therapy sessions scheduled in selected territories. In other psychiatric settings, all interaction between patients and staff (nonmedical as well as medical) may be valued as potentially therapeutic, whether they take place in structured activity settings, or informally, as in corridors or lounges. For this analysis all settings used in any way by patients (other than their own personal territories) should be analyzed either under "therapeutic territories," or under the category "informal spaces."

What areas are considered to be for "therapeutic interaction" between the patients and staff; are these distinct role related activity areas (group therapy room, art therapy studio), or multi-use rooms; or are all areas accessible to patients considered to be potential settings for informal, as well as formal therapeutic interactions? What does this distinction imply about the place of therapy in the larger world of human relations? For each "therapeutic territory," consider the following:

Territory: What is the overt function of this space; what is assumed to be the "therapeutic activity" engaged in by patients and staff? How is the space equipped, furnished and decorated (specialized medical equipment, business-like furniture, nurturing homelike setting, creative imaginative context)? What "basic assumption" is conveyed regarding the manner in which "therapeutic interaction" will take place? What colors, textures, are dominant in this space, and what do they suggest about the tenor of interaction considered appropriate?

Boundary: How is the space enclosed; how permeable (visual, aural) is the boundary between this and adjacent spaces? Do the boundary conditions imply concentrations on the activity, freedom from outside distraction, privacy; or a relationship between this and related activities?

Orientation: How is the furniture arranged in the space, at what distance, and for what kind of social interaction? Do staff and patients have separate or different facilities in the space; is one chair, desk, identified as "staff" territory? What role relationships between patients and staff are suggested by the arrangement of the furniture? Where is this therapeutic setting located in relation to the rest of the hospital; is it centrally located, or distant and inaccessible? What does this suggest about the importance of this activity and its relation to other activities in the hospital? Does the space have large or small windows, and what view is obtained from them; what does this suggest about the relationship of this activity to the outside world, and about appropriate degree of openness to external influence?

2d) Informal Spaces

Note: All areas accessible to patients, and not already considered as "personal" or "therapeutic" territories should be analyzed in this section—lounges, corridors, dining room, recreation room, and so on. What kind of spaces are provided for informal social intercourse among the patients: apart from mingling in lounges and corridors, do they wash, eat, exercise or play together? For each of these common, informal spaces:

Territory: What is the overt function of the space: that is, what is assumed to be the activity that brings patients (and staff?) together informally. How many persons is the space designed for; what facilities, furniture, or provisions are there for what kind of interaction; are there places to sit, formally or informally, at what distance, upright or relaxed; are there places to walk, talk, linger, lean; places to interact intensely, work together? What materials, colors, textures predominate, and what do they suggest is the appropriate manner of interaction?

Boundary: What forms the boundary of this space; is it a visual or acoustic barrier? To what extent does the boundary separate this place, and to what extent does it connect with adjacent areas?

Orientation: How is the furniture arranged; are patients oriented toward each other, or outwards, or toward a central focus? What relationship do the windows and doors provide to other parts of the hospital and to the outside world?

3) PROFESSIONAL STAFF TERRITORIES

For each space (e.g., office) identified as professional staff territory:

Territory: How large is the room, height of ceiling, size of windows? What materials predominate (wood panelling, plaster walls, wood beams)? What are the dominant colors and textures of walls, floor, furniture, fabrics; are they rough or smooth to the touch, visually cool or warm? How is the room furnished (chairs, desk, bookshelves, lamps, rugs); what does the furniture suggest is the most important use of the room? Has the space been personalized with paintings, rugs, plants, photos? What does this territory suggest about the identity or character of its user, their way of relating to others? To what extent is this territory different from patient territories and what does this say about role relationships or status differences?

Boundary: How separate is this place from patient areas; is it on a different floor, separated by doors or corridors? Is it easily accessible to patients? What does this suggest about intended interaction between the staff, when they are here, and the patients? Is it assumed that staff, when here, are available or not? How impermeable is the (visual, aural) boundary of this room, and what does this suggest about the degree of privacy of interaction here?

Orientation: How is the furniture arranged, at what distance apart, and for what type of social interaction; or is attention directed outward to a view? How does the entrance doorway structure the staff member's orientation to the rest of the hospital?

4) NONPROFESSIONAL STAFF TERRITORIES

Of the many nonprofessional staff (nursing aides, kitchen staff), some are identified as having jurisdiction over their own territory. The character of these territories, their relationship to patient areas, are also relevant environmental messages for analysis here.

5) THE HOSPITAL AS EXPERIENCED BY VISITORS

Where do visitors, friends, members of patients' families go when they visit the hospital? Are there particular areas accessible to them and intended for their use? Are these places where staff and patients meet with the visitors; or, for what situations are they intended? For each such space:

Territory: How is this place furnished (chairs, couches, lamps)? What does the setting suggest is the appropriate behavior, attitude?

Boundary: How is the boundary of this space defined and what does it suggest about the assumed relationships between patients, visitors, and staff?

Orientation: How is the furniture arranged, at what distance, and for what kind of interaction?

6) The Patients' Experience of the Larger Community Outside the Hospital

Arrangements are often made for patients to make trips outside the hospital, attend school or university classes, or visit community groups. These arrangements are generally part of a process of reintegrating the patient with the normal everyday world, before the patient is discharged from the hospital. Since these experiences of returning to the outside world are often critical for the patient, their physical context should also be examined in this analysis: these architectural settings may contribute to impressions of the outside world as friendly or hostile, accommodating or austere, totally unrelated to hospital life, or offering some elements of similarity.

7) Background Information

Who made all the environmental decisions (who has control over each of these different environmental messages); who decided on the location of the hospital, who chose the building, who decided what alterations should be made, how the building was to be used, which spaces would be used for which purposes; who decided on interior colors, textures, materials, lighting, furniture and layout? Were these decisions made by an unknown or impersonal governing body, the state commission, or by a known individual?

Appendix 3

A NOTE ON THE SICK ROLE AND A
THERAPEUTIC DOUBLE BIND

Treatment systems exercise social control over persons by regulating access to what Parsons calls the Sick Role. Defining persons as being in need of psychiatric treatment deprives them of options in the pursuit of their lives. At the same time the designation "psychiatric patient" certifies the person's disability status, and legitimizes their withdrawal from social participation and social obligations.

The dysfunctions associated with the assignment of the status of psychiatric patient have been pointed out repeatedly. Once persons are legitimized in that status, treatment systems find it difficult to "unlabel" them and to remove the consequences of that designation. Still, it may be feasible to redefine the implication of the designation, as is attempted in the High Point Hospital treatment program.

In their conception of their patients' illness, and in their view of the constraints imposed upon their patients by that illness, High Point staff exhibit a rather novel, if paradoxical, view of the psychiatric patient sick role. Their instructions and demands place patients into what—following Gregory Bateson's suggestion—we may consider a therapeutic double bind.[1] In the more widely known version of the double bind concept, a patient is placed into a "no win" context, one in which the patient is given what amounts to a "heads you lose, tails you also lose" choice.

However, Bateson also calls attention to the therapeutic potential of the double bind: here patients are placed into an apparently paradoxical context, but one in which they cannot possibly loose. Bateson illustrates one form of such a therapeutic double bind from the work of the gifted psychotherapist Frieda Fromm-Reichman, who treated a young schizophrenic woman who had built up a complex religious delusional system replete with powerful gods. She warned the doctor, at the beginning of treatment, that she had been instructed by her voices not to talk to the doctor. The patient said "God R says I shouldn't talk with you." Dr. Fromm-Reichman replied " . . . to me God R doesn't exist, and that whole world of yours doesn't exist . . . To you, it does . . . So I'm willing to talk with you in terms of that world . . . Now go to God R and tell him that we have to talk and he should give you permission . . . ."[2] As Bateson explains, this paradoxical message represents a therapeutic double bind. Whatever the patient's response—either to deny that the doctor's message can be delivered to God R, or to convey the message and thus become an agent for the demands of the therapist—the outcome can be seen as a gain for the treatment process.

Both destructive and therapeutic double binds may occur in many forms and be conveyed by a therapist or reside in the instructions communicated by a program as a whole.

I suggest that in its conception of psychiatric illness and in their demands on their patients the High Point Hospital program—without explicit recognition—provides an illustration of the use of therapeutic double binds.

The program is committed to what appears to be contradictory positions regarding one, the severity of the psychiatric illness characteristics of their patient population, and two, their patient's ability to meet the requirements of a complex social therapeutic program. On the one hand, hospital ideology dictates that patients are seen as seriously ill and in need of long term treatment—a view that is communicated to patients in many ways. On the other hand, in their everyday interactions with patients, staff also communicate expectations to the contrary. Patients are expected to be able to change, and to be able to meet staff's expectations by engaging appropriately in the variety of behaviors essential to functioning within the quite complex structure of the program.

Thus, patients are subject to seemingly paradoxical perceptions, expectations and instructions. However, the paradox, or bind, is a therapeutic one, since it involves a "reframing" of the sick role in a more hopeful and positive evaluation of the compatibility of psychiatric disorder and social functioning.

Though being defined as seriously ill, patients are, at the same time, defined as capable of learning to live within a complex social environment. With the High Point setting, the patient is instructed that serious psychiatric illness *does not preclude* the acquisition of social skills, deutero-learning and participation in increasingly complex social settings and tasks. If patients adopt this paradoxical conception illness may no longer be incompatible with social learning and functioning within and outside of a treatment setting.

Appendix 4

FINANCING OF PATIENT CARE

Patients are admitted to the treatment program on the basis of their suitability and irrespective of methods of reimbursement.

For example, Medicaid reimbursement policies set a limit of $169.50 per patient day and Medicare provides only $132 per patient day. Nonetheless, one third of the High Point Hospital population are Medicaid patients.

Patient care for the majority of patients is financed by a variety of private insurance plans. Among private insurance plans that finance patient care at High Point Hospital are Blue Cross and Major Medical, Metropolitan Life Insurance, Prudential, Connecticut General, and other insurance carriers. A small number of patients (less than 5 percent in 1984) pay for care from their own funds. The method of financing of patient care in private psychiatric hospitals has undergone major changes since the 1960s. High Point Hospital reflects these trends.

A recent study of High Point Hospital patients found that type of reimbursement had no significant relationship to length of hospital stay and patient condition upon discharge—with the exception of patients who had insurance that limited their stay to 45 days or less (9 percent).

REFERENCES AND NOTES

PART I

Chapter 1

1. Gunderson, J.G., Will, O.A., & Mosher, L.R. (Eds). *The principles and practice of milieu therapy.* New York: Jason Aronson, 1983.
2. Lennard, H.L., & Allen, S. D. The treatment of drug addictions: Toward new models. *International Journal of Addictions,* 1973, *8* (3), 521-535.
3. Lennard, H.L., & O'Briant, R. *Recovery from alcoholism.* Springfield, IL: Charles C. Thomas, 1973.
4. Jansen, E. (Ed.). *The therapeutic community.* London: Croom Helm, 1980.

5. Zubin, J. The role of vulnerability in the etiology of schizophrenic episodes. In J.W. West, & D.E. Flinn (Eds.), *The treatment of schizophrenia*. New York: Grune & Stratton, 1976.

6. While Zubin states the thesis in a particularly lucid form, it has in one version or another been advanced by many investigators. In 1970 I suggested the communicational parameters that may serve as stressors: "Certain qualitative contents of communication are easier to cope with than others. . . . Such difficulties may arise not only . . . from the *quantitative imbalances* in the distribution of given kinds of communication . . . some persons are more vulnerable . . . to negative or destructive communications or less capable of meeting excessive demands. Such vulnerability can be due to differential thresholds for the perception of attacks or demands or to an inability to neutralize them . . . This phenomenon is, perhaps, analogous to an organism's ability to process and neutralize noxious substances to which it has been exposed." Lennard, H.L., & Bernstein, A. *Patterns in human interaction* (2nd ed.). San Francisco, CA: Jossey-Bass, 1970. p. 184

7. Bateson, G. Theory versus empiricism. In M. Berger (Ed.), *Beyond the double bind*. New York: Brunner-Mazel, 1979. pp.234-237.

8. Drury, M. O'C. Conversations with Wittgenstein. In R. Rhees (Ed.), *Recollections of Wittgenstein*. Oxford: Oxford University Press, 1984.

9. Fromm-Reichmann, F. Notes on the development of treatment of schizophrenics by psychoanalytic psychotherapy. *Psychiatry*, 1948, *II*, pp. 263-273.

10. *ibid.*

11. Will, O.A., Jr. Psychotherapy and schizophrenia: Implications for human living. In *Psychotherapy of schizophrenia*, Proceedings of the IVth International Symposium, Turku, Finland, 1971. Amsterdam: Excerpta Medica.

Chapter 2

1. Jones, M. *The therapeutic community*. New York: Basic Books, 1953.

2. Hoffman, H.A. The halfway house as a therapeutic community: A

useful model or a burdensome myth? In E. Jansen, (Ed.), *The therapeutic community*. London: Croom Helm, 1980, pp. 72-85.

3. Hoffman, H.A. *op. cit.*

4. The concept of Therapeutic Work was suggested by the analysis of "Gefuehlsarbeit" or "sentimental work" introduced by Anselm Strauss and colleagues. See, for example, Strauss, A. et al. Gefu ehlsarbeit. *Koelner Zeitschrift fur Soziologie und Sozialpsychologie*, 1980, Heft 4, Westdeutscher Verlag.

5. Goode, W.J. *The celebration of heroes*. Berkeley, CA: University of California Press, 1978, p. 1.

6. Goode, W.J. *op. cit.*

7. Goode, W.J. *op. cit.*, p. 6.

8. Goode, W.J. *op. cit.*, p. 31.

9. Goode, W.J. *op. cit.*, p. 33.

10. Becker, H. Personal change in adult life. *Sociometry* 1964, *27*, pp. 40-53.

11. Becker, H. *op. cit.*

12. Bettelheim, B. *A home for the heart*. New York: Alfred A. Knopf, 1974, p. 42.

Chapter 3

1. Bateson, G. Social planning and the concept of "deuterolearning". *Science, Philosophy and Religion*, Second Symposium, Sept. 2 1942, pp. 81-97.

2. Lennard, H.L., & Bernstein, A. *The anatomy of psychotherapy*. New York: Columbia University Press, 1960, pp.27-28.

3. Fromm-Reichmann, F. Notes on the development of treatment of schizophrenics by psychoanalytic psychotherapy. *Psychiatry*, 1948, *11*, pp. 263-273.

4. Sullivan, H.S. quoted in Will, O.A., Jr. Psychotherapy and schizophrenia: Implications for human living. In *Psychotherapy of schizophrenia*, Proceedings of the IVth International Symposium, Turku, Finland, 1971. Amsterdam: Excerpta Medica.

5. Bettelheim, B. *A home for the heart*. New York: Alfred A. Knopf, 1974.

6. See Chapter 11, Table 11-1.

PART II

Chapter 4

1. Lennard, H.L., & Ransom, D.C. *The therapeutic community: Study of a model*, 1972. (Available from Gralnick Foundation, Port Chester, NY).

2. Lennard, H.L., & Allen, S.D. The treatment of drug addictions: Toward new models. *International Journal of the Addictions*, 1973, *8* (3), 521-535.

3. Lennard, H.L., & O'Briant, R. *Recovery from alcoholism*. Springfield, IL: Charles C. Thomas, 1983.

4. Lennard, H.L., & Bernstein, A. *The anatomy of psychotherapy*. New York: Columbia University Press, 1960.

5. Lennard, H.L., & Bernstein, A. *Patterns in human interaction*. San Francisco, CA: Jossey-Bass, 1970.

6. Lazarsfeld, P.F. Evidence and inference in social research. *Daedalus* 1958, *87* (4).

7. Strauss, A.L., & Glaser, B.G. *The discovery of grounded theory*. New York: Aldine Pub. Co., 1967.

8. Bales, R.F. Preface, *op. cit.*, 4.

9. Barker, R. *The stream of behavior*. New York: Appleton-Century Crofts, 1963.

10. Caudill, W. *The psychiatric hospital as a small society*. Cambridge, MA: Harvard University Press, 1958.

11. Goffman, E. *Asylums*. Garden City, NY: Doubleday, 1961.

12. Stanton, A., & Schwartz, M. S. *The mental hospital*. New York: Basic Books, 1954, p.429.

13. Stanton & Schwartz, *op. cit.* p.448.

14. Lieberman, R. P. Research on the psychiatric milieu. In J.G.

Gunderson, O.A. Will, & L.R. Mosher (Eds.). *Principles and practice of milieu therapy*. New York: Jason Aronson, 1983, p.78.

PART III

Chapter 5

1. I owe a debt to Anselm Strauss and colleagues for their conception of *Gefuehlsarbeit* or sentimental work, introduced in their analysis of activities of medical personnel with chronically ill patients. Their lead in expanding the conception of professional work beyond the traditional analysis of professional roles helped me to formulate the different and perhaps unique conception of therapeutic work that has evolved, over the years, within the High Point Hospital program. See, for example, Strauss, A. et al. Gefuehlsarbeit. *Koelner Zeitschrift fuer Soziologie und Sozialpsychologie*, Heft 4, 1980, Westdeutscher Verlag.
   Strauss, A. et al. *Sentimental work in the technologized hospital*. Dept. of Social and Behavioral Sciences, Univ. of Calif. 1982 (mimeo).

2. From interview with A. Gralnick.

3. *op. cit.* 1.

Chapter 7

1. ". . . the physical setting is . . . taken for granted . . . for any given setting there are countless variations in design and substance that are generally ignored in the attempts to establish the factors that facilitate or hinder the prescribed behaviors." Proshansky, H., Ittelson, W., & Rivlin, L. Freedom of choice and behavior in a physical setting. In H. Proshansky, W. Ittelson, & L. Rivlin (Eds.), *Environmental psychology*. New York: Holt, Rinehart & Winston, 1970, p.173.

   Few studies describe the range of potential therapeutic effects of the physical environment of mental health programs. The most insightful and broadest ranging analysis of therapeutic implications of the built environment can be found in Bettelheim's *A home for the heart.* Bettelheim describes how, in creating a hospital for schizophrenic children, careful attention was paid to environmental messages conveyed by building size, style, and materials, spatial relationships of buildings, size and location of rooms, window details, surface decoration, colors, textures, finishes, furniture design and arrangement. Bettelheim, B. *A home for the heart.* New York: Alfred A. Knopf, 1974.

2. A body of research on the influence of setting on behavior has grown out of the concept of "behavior setting" described in Barker, R. *The stream of behavior.* New York: Appleton-Century Crofts, 1963.

3. ". . . the physical seting is . . . assumed to set the stage for and perhaps define the actors' roles with respect to particular human relationships and activities." Proshansky, Ittelson, & Rivlin, Freedom of choice and behavior in a physical setting. In *Environmental psychology.* New York: Holt, Rinehart & Winston, 1970, p. 173.

On a smaller scale of analysis, Robert Sommer discusses the influence of furniture arrangements on social interaction in mental hospitals in his *Personal space: The behavioral basis of design.* Englewood Cliffs, NJ: Prentice Hall, 1969.

4. ". . . strong considerations should be given to establishing a unit wherein design can promote a patient's sense of security, self-worth, stability and nonconfinement." Planning and design considerations for general hospital psychiatric units. Gershon, H., & Voorheis, H. *Administration in Mental Health,* Spring 1984, *11*(3), 207.

5. It has been argued that "Children internalize not only family relationships and social patterns but also their experience with the nonhuman physical environment". Crowhurst-Lennard, S., The child's conception of built space: An exploratory study. *Education,* Winter 1978, *99*(2), 157-162.

Sivadon's position that "Personality is constituted by the internalization of the organism's successive relations with its environment" leads him to propose that the environment may be considered as a potentially therapeutic modality for psychiatric patients. Sivadon, P. Space as experienced: Therapeutic implications. *Environmental psychology op. cit.,* pp.409-419.

6. Bettelheim discusses in some depth the importance of the character and style of furniture in a children's psychiatric hospital. Bettelheim, *op. cit.*

7. Smith's definition of territory—"encapsulated zones of autonomy" captures the sense of individuality that may be fostered by possession of a territory. Smith, D., Household ecology. Unpublished paper, University of California, Berkeley. c. 1965.

8. "What our experience proves is that, contrary to widespread opinion, comfort and pleasant living aid therapy." Bettelheim, *op. cit.* 1, p.40.

9. Erving Goffman describes how patients in a "total institution" made an effort to maintain their own "personal territory." Goffman, E. *Asylums.* Garden City, NY: Anchor Doubleday, 1961, p. 243.

10. For a detailed discussion of the significance of boundaries see Crowhurst-Lennard, S., & Lennard, H. Architecture: Effect of territory, boundary and orientation on family functioning. *Family Process*, March 1977, *16*(1), 49-66.

11. Corridors have been the subject of many studies, due to their dominant character in most state psychiatric units. Most studies arrive at the conclusion voiced by Sivadon, that "a corridor longer than 40 meters, even if well lit, was anxiety producing if it had no shelters, or better yet, side exits." Sivadon, *op.cit.*5, p. 416.

12. The influence of design on staff-patient role relationships has been often noted. "Territorial behavior is instrumental in the definition and organization of various role relationships. . . . Control of specific territories and the role relationships between people are closely interrelated." Proshansky et al., Freedom of choice and behavior in a physical setting. *op.cit.* 1, p.180.

13. For an analysis of an unusual but effective social model for an alcoholism detoxification center conveyed by a rehabilitated community firehouse, see Crowhurst, S. H. The environment of starting point. Unpublished paper, San Francisco, CA, 1972.

14. Method of construction has seldom been considered in analyses of psychiatric hospitals, though its significance has been marked elsewhere. See Crowhurst-Lennard, S. H. *Explorations in the meaning of architecture.* Woodstock, NY: Gondolier Press, 1980.

15. For a discussion of the significance of building materials, their character, color, texture, and surface finish, see *Explorations in the meaning of architecture, ibid.*

    It has been noted that "... the disturbed patient is often keenly influenced by colors, textures, form, and even spatial arrangements. Indeed we are sometimes dealing with patients whose awareness of their surroundings has a strong influence on shaping behavior and mood." Gershon & Voorheis, *op. cit.*, p.206.

16. The concept of "jurisdiction" is of relevance here. Roos, P. Jurisdiction: An ecological concept. *Environmental psychology, op. cit.* pp. 239-246.

17. This paradigm was originally applied to the analysis of the home. See: Crowhurst, S. H., A house is a metaphor. *Journal of Architectural Education, XXVII*(2,3), 35-53.

18. Goffman, E. *Relations in public.* New York: Harper & Row, 1971, p.63.

19. Lennard, H. L., & Bernstein, A. *Patterns in human interaction.* San Francisco, CA: Jossey-Bass, 1970, pp.158-160.

Chapter 8

1. Gralnick, A. *Humanizing the psychiatric hospital.* New York: Jason Aronson, 1975.

2. To proceed in a systematic way it was necessary to develop an inventory of values that reflected the most salient issues around which patients' day-to-day experiences are organized.

    It was essential that an inquiry into values took a form understandable and acceptable to patients.

    The Value Interview involved two phases: First, patients were asked to look at a series of statements (each placed on a 3" × 5" card) and to indicate whether the value involved (e.g., to be of asistance to others) was of great importance to them, or not too important. They then classified all statements into two sets—of great importance, and not too important.

    However, the patient's initial classification was only the first step in our inquiry. When patients had completed the tasks they were then asked to illustrate, and give examples of the values they consider important. For example, if they consider "being of assistance to others" to be of importance they were asked to provide an example from their everyday life to illustrate the importance of this value to them. Inevitably, in the interview, other priorities emerged and were included in further study.

3. Boszormenyi-Nagy, I., & Krasner, B. Trust based therapy: A contextual approach. *The American Journal of Psychiatry*, July 1980, *137*(7), 761.

4. Berger, P. L. *A rumor of angels.* Garden City, NY: A Doubleday Anchor Book, 1970, p.53.

5. Mayeroff, M. *Caring.* New York: Harper & Row Perennial Library, 1971, pp. 41-42.

6. Mayeroff, W. *op. cit.* 5, p.11.

7. Berger, P. *op.cit.* 4, p.53.

8. Berger, P. *op.cit.* 4, p.61.

9. Frank, J. *Persuasion and healing.* New York: Schocken Books, 1963 p.54.

10. Will, O. A., Jr. Psychotherapy and schizophrenia: Implications for human living. In *Psychotherapy of schizophrenia*, Proceedings of the IVth International Symposium, Turku, Finland, 1971. Amsterdam: Excerpta Medica, p.34.

11. Huizinga, J. *Homo ludens.* Boston, MA: The Beacon Press, 1955.

12. Lennard, H. L., & Bernstein, A. *Patterns in human interaction.* San Francisco, CA: Jossey-Bass, 1970, p.197.

13. Berger, P. L., *op.cit.* 4, p.59.

14. Cousins, N. The anatomy of an illness. *New England Journal of Medicine*, 1976, *259*, pp.1458-1463.

PART IV

Chapter 9

1. McIntyre, A. Patients as agents. In S.F. Spicker, & H.T. Engelhardt, Jr. (Eds.), *Philosophical medical ethics.* Dordrecht, Holland: D. Reidel, 1972, pp.192-212.

2. Boszormenyi-Nagy, I., & Krasner, B. R. Trust based therapy: A contextual approach. *The American Journal of Psychiatry*, July 1980, *137*(7).

3. Gralnick, A. *Humanizing the psychiatric hospital.* New York: The Gralnick Foundation, 1975, p.72.

4. Ramsey, P. *The patient as person.* New Haven, CT: Yale University Press, 1970, pp. XI-XII.

5. Mill, J. S. *On liberty.* London: J. W. Parker, 1859.

6. Jonsen, A. E., & Hellegers, A. E. Conceptual foundations for an ethics of medical care. L. R. Tancredi (Ed.), *Ethics of health care.* Washington DC: National Academy of Science, 1974.

7. Gralnick, A., *op.cit.*, 3.

8. Gralnick, A. Personal communication (taped interview).

9. Boszormenyi-Nagy, I. Ethics of human relationships and the treatment contract. In H.L Lennard & S. Crowhurst-Lennard (Eds), *Ethics of health care.* Woodstock, NY: Gondolier Press, 1980, p.53.

10. Boszormenyi-Nagy, I. *op.cit.*9, p.123.

11. Mayeroff, M. *Caring.* New York: Harper & Row, Perennial Library, 1971, p.79.

12. Foot, P. The problem of abortion and the doctrine of double effect. *Oxford Review*, 1967, *5*,pp. 5-15.

13. Fromm-Reichmann, F. Notes on the development of treatment of schizophrenics by psychoanalytic psychotherapy. *Psychiatry*, 1948, *II*, pp. 263-273.

14. Fromm-Reichman, F. *op.cit.* 13

Chapter 11

1. "The dramatic effect of the short session has been compared by Lacanians to an 'awakening of the patient from a dream-like state'." Schneiderman, S. *Jacques Lacan: The death of an intellectual hero.* Cambridge, MA: Harvard University Press, 1983.

2. Shands, H. *The war with words.* The Hague: Mouton, 1971.

3. The term synergistic has recently been reintroduced into a discussion of social intervention modalities by the family therapist David Mendell who uses it to explain the beneficial changes brought

about in treatment of some patients by the concurrent use of individual, group, and family therapy modalities.

4. Davis, F. Definitions of time and recovery in paralytic polio convalescence. *American Journal of Sociology*, May 1956, pp. 582-587.

5. Roth, J.A. *Timetables: Structuring the passage of time in hospital treatment and other careers*. Indianapolis: Bobbs-Merrill, 1963. One of the virtues of Roth's study is that it is based on both systematic research and personal experience. The sociologist, Julius Roth, spent some time in a TB sanitarium as a patient.

6. Just as the vulnerability to infection continues to characterize the symptom-free TB patient.

PART V

Appendix 1

1. Kraepelin, E. *One hundred years of psychiatry*. New York: The Citadel Press, 1962.

2. Bateson, G. Theory versus empiricism. In M. Berger (Ed.), *Beyond the double bind*. New York: Brunner-Mazel, 1978, p.234.

3. Zola, I.K. Reflecting on directions in psychotropic drug research. In R. Cooperstock (Ed.), *Social aspects of the medical use of psychotropic drugs*. Toronto: Addiction Research Foundation of Ontario, 1974, p.164.

4. Lennard, H.L., & Crowhurst-Lennard, S. *Ethics of health care*. Woodstock, NY: Gondolier Press, 1979, p.3.

5. Will, O.A., Jr. *Psychotherapy*. Presented at the International Conference on Psychoanalysis and Family Therapy, Philadelphia, Oct. 20, 1975. Unpublished lecture.

6. Will, O.A., Jr. Psychotherapy and schizophrenia: Implications for human living. In *Psychotherapy of schizophrenia*, Proceedings of the IVth International Symposium, Turku, Finland, 1971. Amsterdam: Excerpta Medica.

7. Studies have suggested that the prevalence of Tardive Dyskinesia in some hospitalized chronic patient populations treated with neuroleptics is as high as 50 percent. For more conservative esti-

mates of "True" prevalence of Tardive Dyskinesia of 20 to 30 percent see: Kane, J.M., & Smith, J. Tardive Dyskinesia, prevalence and risk factors, 1959–1979. *Archives of General Psychiatry*, 1982, *39*, pp. 473-481, and: Baldessarini, R.J. *Chemotherapy in psychiatry.* Cambridge, MA: Harvard University Press, 1977.

It is difficult to conceive of another medical treatment that results in serious and irreversible side effects in as many as one third of the patients exposed to its long-term use. Yet there is little evidence that there has been a decrease in the use of neuroleptic drugs as the treatment of choice for mental disorder.

8. Fromm-Reichmann, F. Notes on the development of the treatment of schizophrenics by psychoanalytic psychotherapy. *Psychiatry*, 1948, *II*, pp. 263-273.

9. Arieti, S. *Understanding and helping the schizophrenic*, New York: Simon & Schuster, 1980.

10. Lidz, T. *A psychosocial orientation to schizophrenic disorders*. Keynote address to Eighth International Conference on the Psychotherapy of Schizophrenia, New Haven, Oct. 1984.

11. Ciompi, L. Modellvorstellungun zum Zusammenwirken biologischer und psychosozialer Factoren in der Schizophrenie. *Fortschritte der Neurologie-Psychiatrie*, 1984, *52*, pp. 200-206, George Thieme Verlag, Stuttgart.

12. *op. cit.* 5, 6.

13. Gostin, L. *A human condition.* London: Mind, 1977.

14. *Lebensform* can be roughly translated as way of life or mode of being.

15. Bateson, G. *op. cit.*, p. 234.

16. Fromm-Reichmann, F. *op. cit.* 8, p. 179.

17. Lemert, E.M. *Social pathology.* New York: McGraw-Hill, 1951.

18. Scheff, T.J. *Being mentally ill: A sociological theory.* New York: Aldine, 1966.

Appendix 3

1. Bateson, G. et al. Toward a theory of schizophrenia. *Behavioral Science*, 1956, *1*(4), 251-264.

2. *op. cit.* 1., p.264.

BIBLIOGRAPHY

Aricti, S. *Understanding and helping the schizophrenic.* New York: Simon & Schuster, 1980.

Baldessarini, R.J. *Chemotherapy in psychiatry.* Cambridge, MA: Harvard University Press, 1977.

Barker, R. *The stream of behavior.* New York: Appleton-Century Crofts, 1963.

Bateson, G. Social planning and the concept of deuterolearning. *Science, Philosophy and Religion,* Second Symposium Sept. 2, 1942, pp. 81-97.

Bateson, G. Theory versus empiricism. In M. Berger (Ed.), *Beyond the double bind.* New York: Brunner-Mazel, 1978.

Bateson, G. et. al. Toward a theory of schizophrenia. *Behavioral Science,* 1956, *1*(4), 251-264.

Becker, H. Personal change in adult life. *Sociometry*, March 1964, *27*, pp. 40-53.

Berger, P.L. *A rumor of angels*. Garden City, NY: A Doubleday Anchor Book, 1970.

Bettelheim, B. *A home for the heart*. New York: Alfred A. Knopf, 1974.

Boszormenyi-Nagy, I. Ethics of human relationships and the treatment contract. In H.L. Lennard & S. Crowhurst-Lennard (Eds.), *Ethics of health care*. Woodstock, NY: Gondolier Press, 1980.

Boszormenyi-Nagy, I., & Krasner, B. Trust based therapy: A contextual approach. *The American Journal of Psychiatry*, July 1980, *137*(7), 767-775.

Caudill, W. *The psychiatric hospital as a small society*. Cambridge, MA: Harvard University Press, 1958.

Ciompi, L. Modellvorstellungen zum Zusammenwirken biologischer und psychosozialer Factoren in der Schizophrenie. *Fortschritte der Neurologie-Psychiatrie*, 1984, *52*, pp. 200-206, George Thieme Verlag, Stuttgart.

Cousins N. The anatomy of an illness. *New England Journal of Medicine*, 1976, *259*, pp. 1458-1463.

Crowhurst, S.H. A house is a metaphor. *Journal of Architectural Education*, 1974, *XXVII*(2,3), 35-53.

Crowhurst-Lennard, S. H. The child's conception of built space: An exploratory study. *Education*, Winter 1978, *99*(2), 157-162.

Crowhurst-Lennard, S.H. *Explorations in the meaning of architecture*. Woodstock, NY: Gondolier Press, 1980.

Crowhurst-Lennard, S. & Lennard, H.L. Architecture: Effect of territory, boundary and orientation on family functioning. *Family Process*, March 1977, *16*(1), 49-66.

Davis, F. Definitions of time and recovery in paralytic polio convalescence. *American Journal of Sociology*, May 1956, pp. 582-587.

Drury, M.O'C. Conversations with Wittgenstein. In R. Rhees (Ed.), *Recollections of Wittgenstein*. Oxford: Oxford University Press, 1984.

Foot, P. The problem of abortion and the doctrine of double effect. *Oxford Review*, 1967, *5*, pp. 5-15.

Frank, J. *Persuasion and healing.* New York: Schocken Books, 1963.

Fromm-Reichmann, F. Notes on the development of treatment of schizophrenics by psychoanalytic psychotherapy. *Psychiatry*, 1948, *II*, pp. 263-273.

Goffman, E. *Asylums.* Garden City, NY: Doubleday, 1961.

Goffman, E. *Relations in public.* New York: Harper & Row, 1971.

Goode, W.J. *The celebration of heroes.* Berkeley, CA: University of California Press, 1978.

Gostin, L. *A human condition.* London: Mind, 1977.

Gralnick, A. *Humanizing the psychiatric hospital.* New York: Jason Aronson, 1975.

Gunderson, J.G., Will, O.A., & Mosher, L.R. (Eds.). *The principles and practice of milieu therapy.* New York: Jason Aronson, 1983.

Hall, E.T. *The hidden dimension.* New York: Doubleday, 1966.

Hoffman, H.A. The halfway house as a therapeutic community: A useful model or a burdensome myth? In E. Jansen (Ed.), *The therapeutic community.* London: Croom Helm, 1980, pp. 72-85.

Huizinga, J. *Homo ludens.* Boston: Beacon Press, 1955.

Jansen, E. (Ed.). *The therapeutic community.* London: Croom Helm, 1980

Jones, M. *The therapeutic community.* New York: Basic Books, 1953.

Jonsen, A. E., & Hellegers, A. E. Conceptual foundations for an ethics of medical care. In L.R. Tancredi (Ed.), *Ethics of health care.* Washington, DC: National Academy of Science, 1974.

Kane, J.M., & Smith, J. Tardive dyskinesia: Prevalence and risk factors. 1959–1979. *Archives of General Psychiatry*, 1982, *39*, pp. 473-481.

Kraepelin, E. *One hundred years of psychiatry.* New York: Citadel Press, 1962.

Lazarsfeld, P.F. Evidence and inference in social research. *Daedalus* 1958, *87*(4).

Lemert, E.M. *Social pathology.* New York: McGraw-Hill, 1951.

Lennard, H.L., & Allen, S.D. The treatment of drug addictions: Toward new models. *International Journal of the Addictions,* 1973, *8*(3), 521-535.

Lennard, H.L. & Bernstein, A. *The anatomy of psychotherapy.* New York: Columbia University Press, 1960.

Lennard, H.L., & Bernstein, A. *Patterns in human interaction.* San Francisco, CA: Jossey-Bass, 1970.

Lennard, H.L., & Crowhurst-Lennard, S. *Ethics of health care.* Woodstock, NY: Gondolier Press, 1979, p. 3.

Lennard, H.L., & O'Briant, R. *Recovery from alcoholism.* Springfield, IL: Charles C. Thomas, 1983.

Lennard, H.L., & Ransom, D.C. *The therapeutic community: Study of a model.* 1972. Available from Gralnick Foundation, Port Chester, NY.

Lidz, T. *A psychosocial orientation to schizophrenic disorders.* Keynote address to Eighth International Conference on the Psychotherapy of Schizophrenia, New Haven, CT, Oct. 1984.

Lieberman, R. P. Research on the psychiatric milieu. In J. G. Gunderson, O.A. Will, & L.R. Mosher (Eds.), *Principles and practice of milieu therapy.* New York: Jason Aronson, 1983, pp. 67-87.

Mayeroff, M. *Caring.* New York: Harper & Row Perennial Library, 1971.

McIntyre, A. Patients as agents. In S.F. Spicker, & H.T. Engelhardt (Eds.), *Philosophical medical ethics.* Dordrecht, Holland: D. Reidel, 1972, pp. 192-212.

Mill, J. S. *On liberty.* London: J.W. Parker, 1859.

Proshansky, H., Ittelson, W., & Rivlin, L. *Environmental psychology.* New York: Holt, Rinehart & Winston, 1970.

Ramsey, P. *The patient as person.* New Haven, CT: Yale University Press, 1970, pp. XI-XII.

Roth, J. A. *Timetables: Structuring the passage of time in hospital treatment and other careers.* Indianapolis: Bobbs-Merrill, 1963.

Scheff, T.J. *Being mentally ill: A sociological theory.* New York: Aldine, 1966.

Scheflen, A. E. *How behavior means*. New York: Gordon & Breach, 1973.

Schneiderman, S. *Jacques Lacan: The death of an intellectual hero*. Cambridge, MA: Harvard University Press, 1983.

Shands, H. *The war with words*. The Hague: Mouton, 1971.

Sommer, R. *Personal space: The behavioral basis of design*. Englewood Cliffs, NJ: Prentice Hall, 1969.

Stanton, A., & Schwartz, M. S. *The mental hospital*. New York: Basic Books, 1954.

Strauss, A.L., & Glaser, B.G. *The discovery of grounded theory*. New York: Aldine, 1967.

Strauss, A.L. et al. Gefuehlsarbeit. *Koelner Zeitschrift fuer Soziologie und Sozialpsychologie*, Heft 4, 1980, Westdeutscher Verlag.

Strauss, A.L. et al. *Sentimental work in the technologized hospital*. Dept. of Social and Behavioral Sciences, Univ. of California, 1982 (mimeo).

Will, O.A., Jr. Psychotherapy and schizophrenia: Implications for human living. In *Psychotherapy of schizophrenia*, Proceedings of the IVth International Symposium, Turku, Finland, 1971. Amsterdam: Excerpta Medica.

Will, O.A., Jr. *Psychotherapy*. Presented at the International Conference of Psychoanalysis and Family Therapy, Philadelphia, Oct. 20, 1975. Unpublished lecture.

Zola, I.K. Reflecting on directions in psychotropic drug research. In R. Cooperstock (Ed.), *Social aspects of the medical use of psychotropic drugs*. Toronto: Addiction Research Foundation of Ontario, 1974.

Zubin, J. The role of vulnerability in the etiology of schizophrenic episodes. In J.W. West, & D.E. Flinn (Eds.), *The treatment of schizophrenia*. New York: Grune & Stratton, 1976.

INDEX